MIGRAINES and EPILEPSY

MIGRAINES
– and –
EPILEPSY

*How to Find Relief, Live Well,
and Protect Your Brain*

JAMES BOGASH, DC

New York

MIGRAINES and EPILEPSY
How to Find Relief, Live Well, and Protect Your Brain

Published in New York, New York, by Morgan James Publishing. Morgan James and The Entrepreneurial Publisher are trademarks of Morgan James, LLC.
www.MorganJamesPublishing.com

The Morgan James Speakers Group can bring authors to your live event. For more information or to book an event visit The Morgan James Speakers Group at
www.TheMorganJamesSpeakersGroup.com.

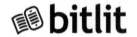

A **free** eBook edition is available with the purchase of this print book.

ISBN 978-1-63047-147-7 paperback
ISBN 978-1-63047-148-4 eBook
ISBN 978-1-63047-149-1 hardcover
Library of Congress Control Number:
2014934762

CLEARLY PRINT YOUR NAME ABOVE IN UPPER CASE

Instructions to claim your free eBook edition:
1. Download the BitLit app for Android or iOS
2. Write your name in **UPPER CASE** on the line
3. Use the BitLit app to submit a photo
4. Download your eBook to any device

Cover Design by:
Rachel Lopez
www.r2cdesign.com

Interior Design by:
Bonnie Bushman
bonnie@caboodlegraphics.com

In an effort to support local communities, raise awareness and funds, Morgan James Publishing donates a percentage of all book sales for the life of each book to Habitat for Humanity Peninsula and Greater Williamsburg.

Get involved today, visit
www.MorganJamesBuilds.com.

Habitat
for Humanity®
Peninsula and
Greater Williamsburg
Building Partner

CONTENTS

INTRODUCTION

The debilitating pain of a migraine. The disability of poorly controlled seizures. If this describes you, or someone you care about, you are not alone. A staggering 3 million people in the United States alone have been diagnosed with epilepsy. When you consider that migraines share very similar characteristics to seizures, you can add another 35 million to the pool. THEN, consider the fact that neurodegenerative disorders, like Parkinson's and Alzheimer's, may be the long-term result of uncontrolled damage to the brain from epilepsy and migraines. This means there are a very large number of people alive today affected by this process that produces a progressive degeneration of the health of our brains.

Most of you have read volumes about your condition and may be as educated, or more so, than the physicians you see for help. This book, unlike others you may have read, will bring together many of concepts that help to heal our brains, improve their function and rid ourselves of debilitating conditions that negatively affect our brains. It is designed as a guide to protect the most important thing you own—your brain. While nothing in the physiology of the brain is guaranteed, the majority of those who follow the recommendations in this book will find relief. Some may be able to rid themselves of migraines or seizures completely.

Before we begin, I need to stress strongly that no information in this book is designed to replace medications you are currently taking. Abrupt withdrawal of anti-seizure or anti-migraine medications can result in dangerous rebound effects, potentially leading to status epilipticus, a life-threatening condition where the brain is locked into a state of perpetual seizure.

With that being said, it is common for mainstream medicine to recommend medications that control the seizure or headache, but do nothing to help protect the brain. This is obviously a severe shortcoming and a grave failing of the way we treat migraines and seizures in society today. It is indescribably important for patients to understand that the ultimate responsibility for their health lies within. It does NOT lie with the physician. Physicians can guide and coach you, but the job of improving the health of your brain is yours alone. It has been shown in research that those who have a higher "health locus of control" have a higher quality of life. In other words, when you believe that the responsibility for your health comes from within, your life, your seizures or your migraines will be better. The bottom line, regardless of all other factors, is that we are in control of our own health. With the exception of a very few purely genetic associations, whatever happens to us is the result of the decisions that we make. Period. We, and not anyone else, are responsible for our health. Many disease states will never be managed effectively until that patient "buys into" the fact that his or her health outcomes depend NOT on their doctor giving them the right medication or surgical procedure, but rather on his or her own choices. Unfortunately much of mainstream medicine does not foster this independent thinking, but rather that a disease is a result of "bad luck" in the genetic lottery and there really isn't anything that can be done, so you have to take this pill. [1]

In general, if we stop a sick neuron from communicating with its healthy neighbor by loading people up with drugs to, in fact, halt their interactive communications, we think we've been successful. All we've done is impede that communication. We haven't fixed the sick neuron. In many cases, that neuron continues to degenerate. If one neuron is going to be sick, it is highly likely there is the environment for other neurons to be sick. So again, taking action to protect your brain is not optional. It is required if you would like to genuinely improve how your brain is functioning and protect your cognitive ability.

The research studies looking at how many people becoming seizure-free show dismal futures for the epileptic patient. I feel that this reflects how inadequate our approaches to seizures and migraines are. We give no advice to help to protect the brain.

Because of that, neurosurgeons are starting to recommend a very scary surgical option for seizures. A recent article actually proposed that 1/3 of epileptic patients are candidates for epilepsy surgery. If a physician recommends surgery with no recommendations for what to do to protect your brain, pack up and run as fast as possible in the opposite direction. To me, the recommendation to take out a portion of your brain and not deal with the problem that started it should be considered malpractice. 2

If the concepts and approaches in this book resonate well with you, follow the principles in it to see how you feel. Give it time – three months, six months or a year – during which time you can continually evaluate how you are feeling. After that time, begin to ask yourself important questions:

- How does my brain respond to stressful situations?
- Are there any breakthrough headaches or seizures I was having before that I no longer am having?
- Is my thinking clearer, and I'm better able to concentrate on important tasks?

Keep your prescribing doctor up to date, explain what you've done and how much improvement you've felt and begin a conversation about potentially adjusting, reducing or eliminating the medications you're on. With that perspective, you can better delve into the root of the problem and manage your condition differently. If your doctor is not willing to work with you on this, FIND A NEW ONE. This is not the type of provider you need for a chronic condition.

In the first chapter, we will begin with a discussion of the differences in some common types of headaches. This is necessary so that headache sufferers can ensure that they have been diagnosed properly. While this chapter does not apply directly to epilepsy, headaches are very common in epileptics, and the following information should be useful.

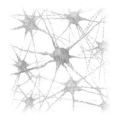

ACCUMULATING SEVERAL TYPES OF HEADACHES

Chapter 1

I t is very common for a patient to have had headaches for many years before seeking help from a chiropractor. Over the years, these patients have accumulated multiple types of headaches. These may be true migraine headaches caused by unhealthy brain cells. They may be structural headaches that will respond very well to treatment from the right type of chiropractor. They may be sinus-related headaches that flare up when environmental or weather conditions change. Or maybe even hypothyroid headaches that are present when you wake up in the morning because that is the time when the thyroid is the least active, resulting in brain cells that do not get enough stimulation from thyroid hormone. All of these have a variety of contributing factors. Unfortunately, unless the treating physician takes a very global approach, the headache patient with multiple types of headaches may get frustrated with care.

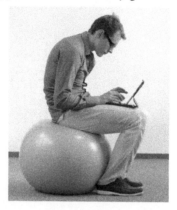

In addition, to have multiple types of headaches over time, it is entirely possible for one type of headache to trigger or make the brain more sensitive to a true migraine. Many headache-sufferers report that a headache may start from stress, skipping a meal, not getting enough sleep or too much time on the computer. But, in a short period of time, that headache is the pathway that triggers a more severe headache that would more appropriately be termed a migraine.

If a headache patient visits a chiropractor and that chiropractor only addresses the articular (joint) component using manipulation, the patient may feel better for an hour or two – maybe a couple of days or even a week. But when the headache comes back, the patient may get frustrated and think that type of approach isn't working. Or the patient may see a massage therapist, and the same pattern occurs. The frustration leads the patient to stop treatment. The patient may then consult a neurologist who may prescribe Imitrex, Topamax,

Neurontin, Depakote or Maxalt, or even Botox injections. And it seems to work for a couple of hours, a couple of days or a couple of weeks only to return in full force. The frustration builds and treatment stops yet again.

It's not until all aspects contributing to a headache are addressed at the same time that the patient can truly achieve the greatest potential for headache relief. That is why it is important to see a physician who will address all potential contributors to a headache, or will work together as a team with other providers. In my own experience, I've had many cases where patients have had headaches for months, years or even decades that were eliminated in two weeks by treating the structural elements. Headaches arising from structural issues are very common, especially in today's high levels of stress and computer use.

STRUCTURAL HEADACHES

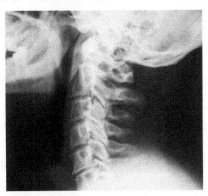

As a chiropractor, I must say that no discussion on headaches would be complete without first addressing the structural component of headaches. A structural headache refers to a headache that is caused by the facet joints of the neck and thoracic region (between the shoulder blades) as well as the soft tissues of the shoulder, neck and head. These soft tissues include muscles, ligaments, tendons and the fascia.

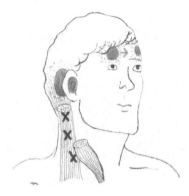

Muscle trigger points and referral patterns

The structural components of this region play a massive, if not the most dominant, role in headaches. This aspect is usually not addressed in an office of a typical neurologist or primary care doctor. It has been a common scenario in my practice to have a patient who has been under the care of a neurologist or a pain management physician for several years, treated only with various medications and procedures without a recommendation to a chiropractor for an evaluation. When the patient finally received comprehensive chiropractic treatment, the treatment relieved the headaches – sometimes in as little as two weeks.

Based on these experiences, I have found that it is far too common for a headache to be diagnosed as a migraine and yet no assessment has ever been done of the joints and soft tissues of this region. I personally think it is impossible to diagnose a migraine without touching the muscles of the neck to ensure this region is not contributing to the patient's headache.[3]

By definition, a migraine occurs on only one side of the head at a time. It can twitch left to right from episode to episode, but a headache that encompasses both sides of the head is not a migraine. That type of headache is most likely structural, and structural care needs to be a component of treatment. Because of that, if you experience structural headaches and it has not been recommended that you see a Doctor of Chiropractic, you may need to find a new doctor who will be open to all treatments for all aspects of your headache.

COMBINING SOFT-TISSUE TREATMENT WITH MANIPULATION

If you're going to seek care from a chiropractor, be certain to consult with one who offers soft-tissue treatment in conjunction with manipulation. The doctor who spends, perhaps, two or three minutes on treatment is not doing you a service. When it comes to headaches, you really need to address the muscles, ligaments, tendons and fascia that overlay the back of the neck, the skull and even the front of the head to truly address what might be contributing to headaches.

BOTOX FOR MIGRAINES?

It is becoming more accepted to use Botox as a treatment for migraines. This approach began as patients who were given Botox injections for aesthetic reasons reported a decrease in their migraine headaches. It is likely that headaches helped with Botox were misdiagnosed and were actually structural in origin. They were stemming from the soft tissues surrounding the eyes such as the temporalis muscle, frontalis muscle and masseter muscles, as well as the fascia that surrounds these muscles. So by giving Botox injections, it was actually relaxing the muscles in that area and relieving the headaches.

PATIENT #1.

Patient #1 had been diagnosed with migraines by her neurologist and put on Topamax. These headaches had been present for a couple of weeks. She really felt they were stemming from the region over the back of her skull and coming up over her head. That is very characteristic of a structural headache. Unfortunately, that pattern wasn't recognized as structural by her neurologist. The Topamax seemed to help with the severity of the headaches, but they were still present. The underlying neck tightness was not addressed at all by the Topamax. Within a matter of a few visits, her headaches started to reduce and the pressure in the neck and the base of the skull started to relax. It is very likely that, ultimately, these headaches will become history.

This particular case gets even more interesting when you examine the most recent medical study probing the effectiveness of Topamax for migraines. The study concluded that Topamax was effective for treating chronic migraines. Based on the abstract, without looking at the study details, a physician may be jumping up and down in excitement thinking, "Wow! Another powerful tool in my arsenal." Yes, Topamax was effective for treating chronic migraines in this study. However, when you take a closer look at the data, over the course of three months, the migraine sufferers had 1.5 fewer headache days during the course of three months. One and a half fewer headache days in three months. That's an average of ½ fewer headache days per month. That was the definition of "effective." The price tag for this level of "effectiveness" was about $600 over the 3 months of the study. Looking back at this patient's treatment, the use of Topamax was doing nothing to actually address or fix the true problem. It was merely masking the symptoms to control some of the headaches in the short term.[4]

Topamax is associated with significant potential side-effects like all the other medications used to treat migraines and seizures such as tingling, fatigue, dizziness, loss of cognitive function and potentially permanent vision changes. In my opinion, using a treatment such as Topamax to provide a mere 1.5 fewer headache days in three months is just sort of worthless and comes with a heavy price tag. If physicians prescribing this drug for headache patients understood the research and said, "If you take this drug, it's got this long list of potential side effects but you're going to have 1.5 fewer headache days in three months," I think most patients would give a quizzical look at the physician and ask, "Don't you have anything more effective?"

The bottom line is any headache-sufferer should see a physician who is going to address all aspects of the problem. In particular, look for a physician who will address the structural aspects of the neck, will combine that with manipulation and will understand the concepts outlined in subsequent chapters.

There are a variety of manual therapies techniques such as fascial manipulation, trigger-point therapy, Active Release Technique, Neuromuscular Re-education or Graston technique. These techniques can be very effective in managing the soft-tissue components of a structural headache. Combine that with manipulation, and the outcomes are going to be much better than they would be with either of those therapies alone.

CHAPTER ONE SUMMARY AND ACTION STEPS

Summary:

1. Multiple headache types of common in long-term sufferers.
2. Having one type of headache may trigger another, more severe headache.
3. Structural headaches stem can stem from the soft tissues of the neck as well as the joints of the neck and upper mid-back and are a very common cause of headaches.
4. Chiropractic care can provide an effective treatment to both the soft tissues and the joints of this region.

Action Steps:

1. If you have not sought the opinion of a chiropractic physician for your headache, make the appointment today. Good referral sources may include:

   a. www.Grastontechnique.com

   b. http://www.facebook.com/pages/Fascial-Manipulation-Workshops/116202938499185?sk=wall

   c. www.triggerpointtherapy.com

   d. www.activerelease.com

   e. www.neuromuscularreeducation.com

2. Keep a daily diary of your headaches for at least one month, if you have not done so already. Identify different patterns:

   a. What triggers your headaches?

   b. What location is it in and does it seems to radiate from a central area?

   c. Do they change locations or character after they start?

   d. What helps to relieve the pain, if anything?

In the next chapter, we will begin to explore the normal process of how our brain cells work. Once you have that understanding, you can better understand how problems begin to occur and how these problems can result in the generation of migraines, seizures and an overall loss of healthy brain functioning

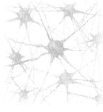

A LITTLE HIGH SCHOOL
BIOLOGY REFRESHER

Chapter 2

ENTER THE MITOCHONDRIA

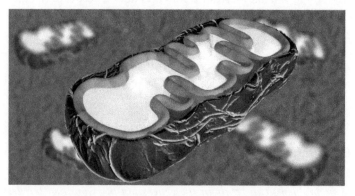

The region of the cell that generates energy

F or background, you need to think way back to your high school biology class and the anatomy of a cell. To the mitochondria. The little "powerhouse of the cell." That little organelle within the cell that helps to generate energy for a cell. And the "energy currency" for every cell is adenosine triphosphate, or ATP. There are some billion or so reactions that occur in our body EVERY SECOND, and each one of these requires a molecule of ATP to get the job done. Some tissues, like fat, use very little energy. Others, like the heart, our muscles and our brain, use much more. At rest, the nervous system, which includes our brain, is the greatest utilizer of ATP in the body. Once we start moving, the muscles take over and have the greatest need.

Imagine that. As you sit here reading this, your brain is requiring mass amounts of energy just to process the information. So what does this mean? It means that each cell of the nervous system requires thousands of mitochondria just to generate the energy needed for a brain cell just to perform its basic functions. And each of these mitochondria are little factories churning out ATP for the brain cell to use at an enormous rate.[5] Evidence has been present for several decades that the protection and nutritional support of the mitochondria needs to be an integral part of avoiding, reducing the severity of and reducing the long-term ramifications of migraines and seizures.[6]

KEEPING THE BALANCE

So, we've decided that neurons require massive amounts of energy in the form of ATP that are generated in the mitochondria. When that process is disturbed, it will begin to fire when it is not supposed to. Too much information begins to be passed from one cell to the other. Again and again and again and again. And again. Too much activity in the brain. Uncontrolled, wild messages passing from cell to cell, continually expanding and catching more and more brain cells in the net of too much activity. A seizure. A migraine.

It would seem that the onset of increased activity, like a seizure and migraine, are actually from TOO MUCH energy, right? Especially a grand mal seizure, with the uncontrolled contractions of the muscles. Or a migraine with high levels of pain. We'll soon find out that the exact opposite is true.

THE PEACEFUL NEURON

To understand this idea better, we need to know some more about how neurons work. A very important aspect of all of our cells is the cell membrane. The cell membrane keeps stuff in that is supposed to stay in and keeps the stuff out that is supposed to stay out. The key players in the neurons are sodium (Na+) and potassium (K+). Levels of sodium outside a nerve cell are about 9 times higher than the levels inside the cell. With potassium, levels inside the cell are about 20 times higher than outside. So, more sodium outside of the cell, more potassium inside the cell.

This essentially creates an electrical charge (for the technical geeks, this is –70 mV) called the resting membrane potential. In a quiet, resting neuron, hovering at this resting membrane potential, there is a natural tendency for the sodium to leak in and potassium to leak out. Luckily, there are pumps in the cell

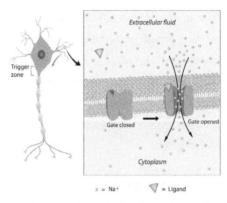

Sodium and potassium moving in and out of cells

membrane that continually maintain this resting membrane potential. These are cleverly called the sodium / potassium pumps (Na+ - K+ pumps). Compare it to a dam that holds back water but has some leaks in it. Water will always try to leak back to the low side of the dam. The installation of a pump on the low side will ensure that the water that leaks out is put back on the high side of the dam. Keep in mind that these sodium potassium pumps require high levels of ATP to continually work to keep sodium out and potassium in. And this is just to keep the cell at rest!

FIRING A NEURON

So, now we have this neuron sitting peacefully, not bothering any of its neighbors. Granted, it is working hard at being peaceful, continually pumping sodium and potassium in and out. When specific circumstances are met, certain gates in the cell membrane will open, allowing some sodium to leak back into the cell. If enough of these sneak back into the neuron (again for the geeks: if enough sodium leaks in to raise the resting membrane potential to the magic number of 55 mV), all heck breaks loose. All the sodium gates open, allowing sodium to rush in, swinging the charge of the neuron into the positive range, and firing off the neuron. This firing of a neuron results in the release of a compound called a neurotransmitter from the tail end of the cell.

NEUROTRANSMITTERS AND "POP A SHOT"

In order for the brain to function, the brain cell needs to be able to pass a message from one cell to another. The problem is that neurons do not directly connect to one another. Instead, they are separated by an opening called the synaptic cleft. In order for a message to pass from one neuron to another, the message must be "tossed" across this synaptic cleft. Neurotransmitters are the "containers" that carries messages across the cleft. There are many neurotransmitters with names like serotonin, GABA (gamma-aminobutyric acid), glutamate, epinephrine, norepinephrine, dopamine and PEA (phenylethylamine), just to name a few. I envision the entire process like a miniature "pop a shot" game. The ones with the small basketball that you have to throw through the hoop as many times as possible before the timer runs out. The basketball is the neurotransmitter. Every time it goes through the hoop, the "message" has made it from one neuron to the next. Give yourself more balls to throw and you have a better chance of getting this message across. This is how drugs like Prozac work—by keeping the basketball (in this case the neurotransmitter serotonin) in play longer by keeping it in the synaptic cleft for a longer period of time. It does not, however, increase the number of balls available. It just keeps them in the cleft longer. Natural compounds like 5-HTP (5-hydroxytrytophan) can work by giving the neuron more serotonin to work with, thereby increasing the number of basketballs and increasing the likelihood that the message will get passed on.

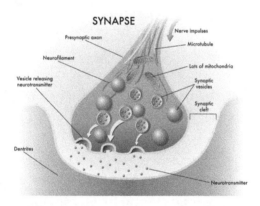

SYNAPSE

A brain cell communicating with its neighbor

CHAPTER TWO SUMMARY AND ACTION STEPS

Summary:
1. The mitochondria are a critical part of the functioning of a healthy cell.
2. It requires a tremendous amount of energy, in the form of ATP, for a cell of the nervous system to function properly.

3. The cell membrane of a brain cell is designed to keep sodium ions out of and potassium ions in the cell.
4. A brain cell fires when this switches, and sodium ions flood across openings in the cell membrane and end up inside the cell instead of on the outside.
5. Brain cells use compounds called neurotransmitters to pass a message from one cell to its neighboring cell.

Action Steps:
1. Reread this chapter to better understand the basics of how a brain cell works.
2. Continue to reread this chapter until you can confidently request the Jeopardy category of "Normal Functioning of a Neuron for $500, Alex."

In Chapter 3, we will begin the process of looking at how the lifestyle factors we choose to adopt influence the ability of our neurons to generate the energy needed to function at an optimum level.

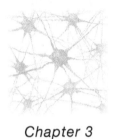

FREE RADICALS AND OXIDATIVE STRESS

Chapter 3

FREE RADICALS

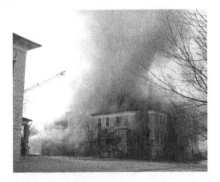

Here's the catch in the way a neuron works. It requires a massive amount of energy (in the form of ATP). You can't make all this energy needed to run a healthy neuron

17

without waste by-products. Imagine lighting a fire to cook or heat water. When you do this, smoke is going to be produced as a by-product of the fire. And we all have heard that in a house fire, more victims die of smoke inhalation than from the fire itself. So this smoke can be dangerous. In physiology, this "smoke," produced as a by-product of generating ATP, is termed "free radicals."

You may have heard of free radicals before. These free radicals are hostile little molecules that damage anything they touch. For those of you who used to play with fireworks as a child, the little "buzzing bee" type of firework always reminds me of a free radical. When they were lit, these little fireworks started to spin very rapidly in a circle, faster and faster, spitting small flames out the side. The end result is a small circle of fire spinning and buzzing all over the ground. So, picture this little buzzing bee molecule bouncing around inside of your cell, damaging anything it touches. Proteins in the cell, your DNA, even the mitochondria that produces the free radicals in the first place while making ATP. All can be damaged by free radicals.

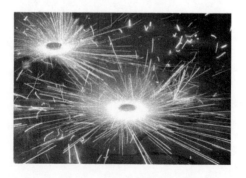

So, the mitochondria in our cells produce the valuable ATP to give each and every cell the energy it needs to get stuff done. However, the side-effect of producing ATP generates potentially dangerous by-products called free radicals. These free radicals have the potential to damage everything in their path. Left unchecked, they can damage the cell's genetic material, leading to cancer. They can damage other components of the cell, leading to buildup of waste materials and poorly performing cells. They can even damage the very mitochondria that are producing the ATP and free radicals. Complicating this bad situation is the fact that the mitochondria do not do a very good job of protecting themselves from free radical damage. So the one part of the cell that we really, really want to protect and keep from being damaged can't really protect itself very well. Too much damage and the mitochondria itself dies off, leaving the poor little neuron with fewer ATP factories to run the way it's supposed to.

OXIDATIVE STRESS

So what happens when the production of these free radicals exceed our cell's ability to protect against them? We develop a condition called oxidative stress. So what causes oxidative stress? In today's processed society, there are almost countless things that contribute to oxidative stress. First and foremost is diet. Eating heavily processed foods low in phytonutrients (we'll discuss phytonutrients in chapter 4) is well known to increase the amount of oxidative stress that our bodies and brains have to respond to. Another major contributor to oxidative stress that many people are not even aware of is oxidative stress caused by our environment.

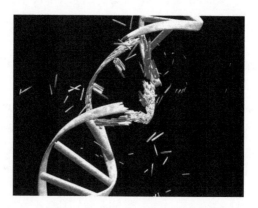

Free radicals can damage DNA

ENVIRONMENTAL CHEMICALS

There is a barrage of more than 82,000 chemicals registered with the FDA that we are exposed to on a daily basis. This ranges

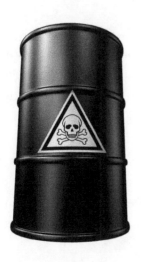

from having your house sprayed for bugs, sprayed for weeds, to all the pesticides, fungicides and herbicides that are used on our conventionally grown produce. It needs to become a matter of looking around. We have tens of thousands of chemicals in our environment that we were never exposed to before, that our bodies are unsure of how to process and eliminate. As an example, there are the flame retardants built into things like clothing, mattresses, pillows, dog beds and furniture. As a matter of fact, as of July 2007, mattresses have had a much higher level of flame-resistance than before that date, and the amount of chemicals required to make it that flame-resistant are much higher. These chemicals actually show up in our bloodstream and may contribute to health problems like infertility.[7] Another example is the use of nonstick cooking surfaces. This surface is achieved through the use of chemicals that also show up in the bloodstream and contribute to oxidative stress.

ARTIFICIAL SWEETENERS

It's also artificial sweeteners. Aspartame is well known to cause the cells of the brain to run faster, sort of like a hamster on a wheel. As the hamster runs on the wheel, going faster and faster and faster, it starts to create much more oxidative stress on the brain. It does this through partial conversion to the neurotransmitter aspartic acid. Aspartic acid is one of those neurotransmitters that drives the neurons to go faster and faster. This is the compound that many researchers use on animals to create seizures so they can test the effectiveness of anti-seizure drugs.

HEAVY METALS

Technically, to the high school chemistry professor, a "heavy metal" is a compound that has a very high density and would be found toward the end of the periodic table of elements. The term "heavy metal," when it pertains to health, however, refers to any molecule that can have a negative effect on the human body such as lead, cadmium, arsenic and mercury.

Many heavy metals to which we are exposed contribute to oxidative stress: cadmium in cigarette smoke or lead, arsenic, antimony and mercury in manufacturing. Mercury is one of the most potent neurotoxins on the planet. Eating fish, primarily wild caught fish that are carnivorous, like ahi, mahi, sharks and halibut, can be a large contributor to our body's burden of mercury. What happens is that mercury, naturally present in our environment as well as the mercury from manufacturing, manages to make its way into the water. From the water, the vegetarian fish like salmon, trout and cod absorb small amounts mercury in their systems. However, when these fish are eaten by other fish, the fish cannot get rid of mercury effectively. Thus, the mercury continues to build up and build up in their bodies. This is referred to a "bioaccumulation." So, carnivorous, older fish -- the ones eating the other fish with lower levels of mercury -- have higher levels of mercury. The older fish have higher levels because they have had more time to bioaccumulate, so albacore tuna has higher levels of mercury than white tuna because it's an older fish.[8]

Lead is another heavy metal that is present in our environment and increases the levels of oxidative stress in the body. It has the ability to interfere with the amount of oxygen we can deliver to the brain. Less oxygen to the brain means less energy and ATP formation. Now that lead- and mercury-based paints have been phased out of use, our principle source of exposure to lead is from lead-contaminated dust particles that travel into our homes from our shoes and clothing, although you might want to properly dispose of that 20-year old can of paint buried in the back of the garage. That calls for you to leave your shoes, coated with lead dust, outside the door when you come home.

STRESS

Another cause of oxidative stress is emotional stress. Stress plays a major role in how efficiently our brain functions. Emotional stress is well known to increase the amount of oxidative stress that the brain experiences. Stress will be covered in much greater detail in the chapter on hormones.

REDUCING THE OXIDATIVE LOAD

So, what do we do to start to reduce the amount of oxidative stress that our bodies and our brains are exposed to? Well, obviously we start with diet. This means avoiding processed foods. I have what I refer to as my "8-year-old" rule. If a typical 8-year-old cannot read the ingredients, it probably means we shouldn't be eating it. Unfortunately, a lot of foods these days won't pass the "35-year-old biochemist" rule. I remember looking at a "food" item from one particularly large manufacturer of food products. Normally when I look at the ingredients, I can get an idea from where the chemicals may be derived. In this particular case, I had no idea (the ingredient was azodicarbonamide) - it wasn't until I looked it up on the Internet that I discovered that it is actually a derivative from the petroleum industry. This is in our FOOD!! So, we need to rid ourselves of the processed chemicals in our food. This means living as organic as possible. Environmental Working

Group (www.ewg.org) is a phenomenal resource for the pesticide levels in produce. They have a list called the "Dirty Dozen" and the "Clean 15." These are list of the produce most likely to contain pesticides and produce least likely to contain them. So, obviously, if you are eating something on the Dirty Dozen list, you want to make sure that you go either locally grown or organically grown whenever possible. On the flip side, it becomes less important, from the pesticide standpoint, when you're dealing with fruits and vegetables on the Clean 15 list.

Another must for decreasing levels of oxidative stress is increasing the intake of high phytonutrient foods. Phytonutrients are all the brilliant colors and flavors and scents found in nature that we will talk about shortly. It is making sure that 95 percent of the food that crosses your lips has high phytonutrient levels that have not been processed out. This needs to be combined with a lower caloric intake. The more calories we have, the more it fuels the fire and the more free radicals we have and the more oxidative stress that our bodies have to deal with. So cutting back on calories after you've begun to increase the levels of phytonutrient-rich foods will lower the levels of oxidative stress your brain has to manage. Maybe it means sharing a meal. Maybe it means preparing less food and not having leftovers. It seems like whenever there's more food, people eat more. There's nothing wrong with not having anything left over because you didn't make quite as much as you normally do.

Exercise is another great way to lower the levels of oxidative stress. Exercise is well known to protect the brain. When you look at studies on depression and anxiety, exercise is one of the most powerful tools we have to manage brain health.

Again, it means decreasing the amount of chemicals in our environment. That means NOT having your house sprayed for bugs. This is not always easy. I remember when we had an ant infestation and ants were making it over to the dog bowl. My 3-year-old, a 10-year-old and I took duct tape and used it to pick up all the ants that kept coming into the house for the next several of days. In the meantime, grits were used to destroy the queen and send the ants elsewhere. (The ants took the grits back to the queen where they are ingested. Unable to release the gas that built up as the grits expanded, the queen died). I occasionally have to battle cockroaches in the house, but it's a much better alternative than having my family exposed to a barrage of chemicals and compromising their long-term health. It also means that my dogs are not exposed to chemicals because we are not spraying the ground where they live.

BENEFITS OF OXIDATIVE STRESS

I know we have only covered oxidative stress as a bad thing. However, as with anything else, the true answer lies somewhere along the spectrum between extreme oxidative stress and none. Much like the organic veggies producing protective compounds in response to stress, our bodies will actually upregulate our production of protective enzymes in response to stressors. A perfect example is our very own white blood cells (WBCs). When faced with an invader, these cells rush to the site of invasion and engulf their enemies. But to destroy the little critters, be they parasites, viruses or bacteria, the

WBC produces high amounts of very concentrated hydrogen peroxide, which very little organic matter can withstand. So our bodies actually use oxidative processes to protect us from infection. If we were to completely block all oxidative stress in our bodies, it is likely we would not be able to fight off an infection or remove cellular debris after an injury. Oxidative stress is also known to begin a process of activating certain genes to produce more of our body's own antioxidant enzymes. This becomes a very strong factor in our body's ability to stand up and fight against free radicals.

CHAPTER THREE SUMMARY AND ACTION STEPS

Summary:

1. Free radicals are created as a by-product of generating energy for a cell.
2. Free radicals have the potential to damage everything in its path.
3. When the number of free radicals exceeds our body's ability to protect against them, we have a dangerous situation called "oxidative stress."
4. Oxidative stress can be created by many factors:
   a. Chemical toxins from the world around us.
   b. Artificial sweeteners like sucralose and aspartame.
   c. Heavy metals.
   d. Stress, both psychological and physical.
5. We can protect against oxidative stress in many ways:
   a. Following the "8-year-old rule" to eat less processed foods, buying organic when possible.

b. Increase the phytonutrient levels of our diet while beginning to cut back on the amount of calories we take in.

c. Exercise.

d. Avoid chemical exposure as much as possible.

Action Steps:

1. Never buy anything without reading the label. Better yet, buy foods that don't need to come with a label. Do not buy food items that contain ingredients you cannot pronounce without embarrassing yourself in a crowd of chemistry students.

2. Switch your shopping away from the big commercial grocery stores to smaller, healthier farmer's markets.

3. Print out a copy of the "Dirty Dozen" list and keep it with you. For items on this list, try to buy organic if possible.

4. Avoid ALL artificial sweeteners like the plague.

5. Examine sources of chemical exposures in your life and reduce when possible:

a. Plastic water bottles and food storage containers.

b. Cosmetic and beauty products (to include hair dye).

c. Household cleaning products.

d. Pesticides, herbicides, insecticides, fertilizers.

e. All exposure to cigarette smoke.

f. Old cushions or other compounds that are flame-resistant.

g. Mattresses made after July 2007.

      h.   Airborne particles (use a room air cleaner).

      i.   Sign up to receive updates from www.EWG.org.

In Chapter 4, we will begin to look at how to protect our brains from the barrage of oxidative stress that our neurons experience, using diet and targeted nutritional supplementation

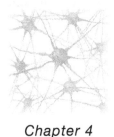

PROTECTION FROM FREE RADICALS

Chapter 4

R emember that oxidative stress is the situation where our cell's ability to quench the free radicals constantly being produced is not strong enough and where free radicals begin to escape, causing damage to everything in their path. While reducing oxidative stress is important, it's akin to the analogy of closing the barn door after the animals have stampeded out. The key is to keep the situation under control in the first place. This involves making sure we have full protection against those nasty free radicals.

Given the high demand of energy that our brain cells require, our brain cells are particularly susceptible to damage from oxidative stress.[9]

Luckily, given the brilliance of the design of the body, we already have protection built in. Thousands of compounds in nature, as well as compounds produced by our body, help fight off free radicals. Let's start with the basics. They fall into three main categories: antioxidants, internally produced enzymes and phytonutrients.

ANTIOXIDANTS

We are all familiar with the term "antioxidant." Vitamin C. Vitamin E. CoEnzyme Q10 (or CoQ10). Alpha lipoic acid. These are just a few of the vitamins that we know have a direct antioxidant effect by attaching themselves to the free radical, thus essentially quenching the smoke and its potential damage. So, in many cases, direct intake of certain antioxidant vitamins can help lower the amount of free radical damage. However, this is where things can get a little tricky. Most of us know that there are fat-soluble (A, D, E and K) and there are water-soluble (the Bs, C) vitamins. We need a balance between these. What if a vitamin like Vitamin E is floating around in a fatty membrane and grabs ones of these free radicals — just wraps its loving little vitamin arms around the damaging free radical. Well, this free radical is actually somewhat contagious. If the Vitamin E hangs onto the free radical long enough, the Vitamin E "catches fire" and can do the same damage that the free radical was intent on causing. Remember that the Vitamin E is fat-soluble and cannot just leave the cell membrane whenever it wants to. So it's essentially stuck there, holding onto the hot potato that is the free radical. The Vitamin E needs something water-soluble that can come and grab the hot potato. Along comes the water-soluble antioxidants like Vitamin C to grab the hot potato and move it away for further processing. So, it is ultimately about balance. We cannot overdose ourselves on a single antioxidant and hope for the best outcome. It is likely that this approach can result in MORE damage than we set out to protect from.

INTERNALLY PRODUCED ENZYMES

Internally produced enzymes have long names like superoxide dismutase and glutathione peroxidase that would leave your opponents in Scrabble drooling with envy. But these enzymes are arguably our most potent defenders against the evils of free radicals. What is interesting is that our diets can actually regulate how much of these enzymes we produce. Certain compounds in the foods and spices we eat, like the carnosol in rosemary, the turmeric in curry and mustard, compounds in green tea and cinnamaldehyde in cinnamon, can actually work their way down from our stomachs to the very vault of DNA in the depths of our cells. From there, these very compounds can sit on our DNA and turn segments of it on or off. That is a powerful way to look at our foods. We've gone so far down the dark path of nutrition that many times the value of our meals is boiled down to their macronutrient construction: 25% carbs, 50% protein, 25% fat… What an awful way to look at our food. BUT, if we look deeper into the compounds that make up the foods we eat, we can envision our food sending little messengers to the heart of what makes up each of us– our DNA. So, as we stare at our next mega-sized value meal, we must think carefully about what message is being sent. Compare that to a beautifully adorned meal vibrant with all the colors, scents and flavors Mother Nature provided and its messages.

PHYTONUTRIENTS

Now we come to the class of compounds called phytonutrients. They have exotic names like flavanoids, bioflavanoids, polyphenols and catechins. There are thousands upon thousands of them known, and we discover new ones every year. In nutrition today, we look at the importance of food based on its vitamin and macronutrient content. How much fat? How much fiber, carbs or protein? Does this have enough Vitamin C to keep me from getting scurvy? How about enough D to keep osteomalacia or rickets at bay? Pellagra? Beriberi? This is how we rank our lunches for kids. I remember talking to one of the nutritionists for a local school district about my son's poor lunch quality. He went on to assure me that the food exceeded federal guidelines for saturated fat, Vitamin C and fiber. Great. So the kids won't get scurvy. I can sleep at night. But what about the thousands of compounds processed out of our diets? Have those been meticulously cataloged and replaced back into the lunch meal? How about into that value meal? When we pull up the nutrition facts that so many of us live by, do we see pages and pages and pages on the fries alone detailing not only the folic acid and Vitamin C content, but which polyphenols are still present? Of course not. They're no longer found in the processed and packaged foods we eat in this the U.S.

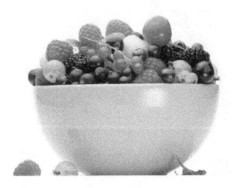

So going back to an unprocessed diet rich in phytonutrients is of utmost importance. Foods like quinoa, honey, broccoli, brussel sprouts, brewed coffee, dark chocolate, deeply colored berries, artichokes, spices, walnuts and pecans are loaded with these protective compounds. Study after study have shown that they will directly protect your mitochondria from free radicals as well as providing indirect protection by telling your DNA to make even more protective enzymes.

GREENS DRINKS

Over the past few years, an increasing number of "greens" type drinks have become available on the market. These are phytonutrient rich drinks composed of things like alfalfa, kale, blue green algae and other long lists of stuff like that. While nothing will ever compare to the broad array of compounds in the foods themselves, if financially feasible, the addition of these drinks to a good quality lifestyle can only be beneficial. I do have to add a few caveats, though, because the quality of these drinks varies widely. First, absolutely, positively NO ARTIFICIAL SWEETENERS!! We will delve into this later. Secondly, if possible, you need to determine whether the drink you're looking at is highly alkaline. Our bodies and our cells function much better when bathed in an alkaline environment. In an alkaline greens drink, most of the minerals, like potassium, are still present in the mixture. A greens drink should also be made of non-GMO materials. GMO stands for "genetically-modified organisms" and has been increasingly, quietly introduced into our food supply. Look for GMO-free certified or organic labels. Finally, since products like blue-green algae can be contaminated with heavy metals if grown improperly, the product should be independently tested to be free of contaminates and heavy metals. This type of certification will be proudly proclaimed on the label.

ORGANIC VS CONVENTIONAL

While we're on the subject of foods rich in phytonutrients, we have to have a discussion on organic versus conventional foods. We generally think of organic produce having less pesticide residues (which is true). However, less thought is given to the produce's phytonutrient content. These plants don't make these compounds for the nice humans to come along and eat them and live happily and healthily ever after. Absolutely not!! These compounds are metabolically expensive to make, and plants are only going to make them if they have a reason. These protective phytonutrients act as natural anti-fungals, anti-parasitics, sunscreens, attractants for insects and animals, anti-bacterials... You get the idea. Plants are making these to protect themselves from their own environment and to survive. Now what happens if we artificially alter the plants' environment with chemical fertilizers, chemical anti-fungals, chemical anti-bacterials, chemical anti-parasitics and shade them? I envision a buff, healthy looking vegetable lifting weights on the organic side, with a slovenly, uncaring vegetable sitting under a beach umbrella sipping a drink with an umbrella in it. Which one is going to have a higher number of healthier compounds? Of course! The buff, organically grown veggie. As an example, we have seen that tomatoes grown organically have higher levels of the red pigment lycopene, which has been shown to help protect the prostate from prostate cancer, than its conventionally grown counterpart. Then add a dose of extra pesticides, and the choice becomes clearer.

SUMMARY OF PROTECTION

So, overall, our body's production of its own antioxidant protection (endogenous), coupled with antioxidants from a broad array of compounds from the foods and spices we consume, can create a balanced protection against free radicals. Balance between the types of antioxidants is equally as important. Some, like Vitamin C, are water-soluble. Others, like Vitamin E, are fat-soluble. Other still have characteristics of both, like alpha lipoic acid. So what happens if a fat-soluble molecule, like Vitamin E, grabs a free radical roaming by? That Vitamin E cannot hang onto the free radical indefinitely. The fat-soluble molecule cannot leave the cell membrane to bring that nasty little free radical to where it needs to go for disposal. In swoops a water-soluble antioxidant like Vitamin C to grab that free radical and transport it away. Much like a molecular baton race. Without this balance, the Vitamin E will soon catch fire and become its own fireball of oxidative stress.

So…we've covered, in far more detail than you've probably ever wanted, the concept of mitochondria, oxidative stress, free radicals and phytonutrients. As exciting as these concepts are, I'm sure you're going to want to go back and read the information again until you've got it down pat. If you understand these concepts, you will have a much better understanding of what happens when brain function starts to go all screwy. I call this situation "sick neurons."

CHAPTER FOUR SUMMARY AND ACTION STEPS

Summary:

1. Antioxidants are compounds like Vitamin C, Vitamin E and CoQ10 that protect against the damage that free radicals can cause.

2. Our bodies have the ability to produce enzymes that strongly protect against free radical damage.

3. Thousands of plant-based compounds, called phytonutrients, are strong protectors against free radical damage.

4. "Greens drinks," which are typically powdered drink mixes containing a broad mix of protective, bland-based compounds, may be a great addition to aid your body in fighting off free radicals.

5. Organic produce contains higher levels of phytonutrients and lower levels of pesticides.

Action Steps:

1. Add a base of antioxidant supplements:
   a. Vitamin C @ 2,000 mg / day.
   b. Vitamin E (as mixed tocopherols) @ 200 IU / day.
   c. CoQ10 @ 50-200 IU / day (depending on how much you can afford).
   d. Alpha Lipoic Acid @ 400 mg / day.
   e. Add a daily scoop of a greens drink.
2. Buy organic when possible
3. If you are not currently exercising, begin today. Start with 20 minutes of walking, 10 push-ups and 10 sit-ups.

In Chapter 5, we will begin to look at what happens to our neurons when levels of oxidative stress rise within our body. This rise in oxidative stress leads to sick neurons, and sick neurons lead to seizures and migraines

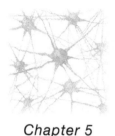

Chapter 5   **SICK NEURONS**

W e've learned that free radicals can begin to destroy the cell from the inside out, starting with the mitochondria. Consider that a typical neuron may contain thousands of mitochondria. The reason the neuron has so many mitochondria is because it requires massive amounts of energy to keep that little sodium ion and that little potassium ion on their proper sides of the cell membrane. So what if a neuron begins to lose more and more of these valuable mitochondria though free radical damage? Eventually, the brain cell cannot produce enough ATP to drive those sodium pumps.[10] This becomes a very serious problem. Remember that we HAVE to keep moving those sodium ions back out of the cell because the darn things keep leaking back in. If we can't control the leakage, the neuron can't keep itself at peace and will fire before it is supposed to. It fires spontaneously because it doesn't have the energy needed to stop it from firing.

So, in the above scenario, this neuron becomes sick because of the damage to its mitochondria and will then fire when it's not supposed to. This causes the release of a neurotransmitter to the next cell, which causes THAT cell to fire when it's not supposed to. And so on, and so on, and so on. Our brains also have a type of neuron called an inhibitory interneuron. The only job of this guy is to stop other neurons from firing. It fires just to keep other neurons from firing. Kind of like a teacher in the front of a classroom constantly "shushing" the rambunctious students. If she stopped shushing, the entire class would erupt into talking. So what happens if this type of brain cells begins to get sick and can no longer fire and thus can no longer "shush" its neighbors? Pandemonium. This uncontrolled firing of whole regions of neurons can generate a seizure or the beginnings of a migraine. All of this because the mitochondria was no longer able to supply the energy needs of the cell.

Uncontrolled firing of all the brain cells starts to burn out these cells. They keep getting the message to fire again and again and again. This places more and more of a demand for ATP on these cells, perpetuating the cycle of destroying the mitochondria and the cell's ability to only fire when it is supposed to fire.

As mentioned before, one of the neurotransmitters that causes brain cells to go crazy is called glutamate. There is no doubt that more of this excitatory neurotransmitter will drive our neurons faster and faster. It turns out that oxidative stress may destroy the transporters that pick up glutamate from outside of the cells, leaving this neurotransmitter to keep sending its message again and again and again—constantly sending the neuron into overdrive.[11]

If the neurons lose too many of their own mitochondria through this process, ultimately the remaining mitochondria can no longer keep up with the energy of the cell, and the cell begins a process called apoptosis, or cell suicide.[12,13] If you can envision a solid Scottish accent and can picture Scotty from Star Trek calling up to the bridge, say, "Captain, we can hold 'er together anymore," then you get an idea of what begins to happen (except Captain Kirk always seems to figure out the problem and save the U.S.S Enterprise—not so much in our brains at this point.).

Left unchecked, this loss of neurons over the course of years can lead to other neurological conditions like Alzheimer's or Parkinson's.[14,15,16,17,18]

CHAPTER FIVE SUMMARY AND ACTION STEPS

Summary:

1. Free radical damage to our cells begins to destroy the mitochondria.

2. When mitochondria are destroyed, the neuron actually fires more.

3. When a neuron fires more, the entire brain becomes overactive, leading to migraines and seizures.

4. Eventually the cell cannot survive this abuse and they begin to die off.

Action Steps:

1. The steps outlined in the following chapters will help to protect the process by which your brain cells function and remain healthy.

2. These steps are NOT optional. Understand, that if you are reading this book because you have migraines or seizures, your neurons are already sick. This process will continue if you keep doing the same things you have been doing.

3. Pay careful attention to the remaining chapters. As you read, consider how you can integrate these concepts into your life.

In Chapter 6 we will look at how powerful exercise is at protecting our brains. In addition, we will cover the types of exercise that will give you the most bang for your buck in protecting the brain.

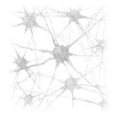

Chapter 6   **EXERCISE**

I n this chapter, we are going to talk a little bit more about exercise. The first thing to understand is that exercise, or rather not exercising, is not an option. Our bodies were designed for heavy physical activity, and our ancestors likely had to work their butts off just to survive. There was no remote control on the TV. Heck, there was no TV. There was no car. There was none of today's amenities. Everything had to be done by manual labor, and that is much more akin to what our bodies are programmed for.

I see a lot of patients who do not exercise and do not really have much of an interest in exercising, but there is a price to be paid. I don't understand how those people think they can get away with not exercising. Without a doubt, a lack of exercise is going to dramatically reduce their quality of life, if not today, then in the future. That being said, let us move on to what I consider some of the best approaches to exercising.

AEROBIC EXERCISE

Let's start with aerobic type activity. I believe that the human body was much more attuned for short-burst aerobic activity rather than the typical 45-plus minutes of continuous exercise. If you think about it, name an animal that we could either chase or would chase us for 40 or 45 or 50 minutes and we'd stand a chance of surviving or catching. We are not going to outrun a saber-toothed tiger for 40 minutes, nor are we are going to chase down an antelope for 40 minutes. I just don't think that, from an evolutionary standpoint, our bodies were designed for long-term aerobic activity. The medical research increasingly favors and supports short-burst aerobic type activities. I can envision us in a hunter-gatherer society, hiding out in a bush. All of a sudden, we would have to jump out and attack an animal or throw our spear or a rock at whatever we happen to be trying to hunt at that time. I think that our bodies are well attuned to these types of actions.

We also know, from a cardiovascular standpoint, that the faster our heart rates come back down to normal after exertion, the better our cardiovascular health. Thus, the idea of short-burst aerobic type activity really strengthens this association. There is a doctor who developed the PACE program (that is the Progressive Accelerating Cardiopulmonary Exertion program), and its premise is much like interval training, but with each interval successively more intense, but shorter. This is easily adaptable to anything that you would want to do. Running, jogging, jump roping, eliptical, swimming -- anything can be done with these concepts in mind.

There was a study done with a group of sedentary young men. All they did (you might want to get your calculators out for this one) were 30-second bursts on an exercise bike, going as fast as they could go. They did that for 4-6 sets, 3 times a week, for 2 weeks. For those of you good with math, this is 9 minutes a week of short-burst aerobic exercise. Astoundingly, they saw a 23% improvement in the way insulin was working in the human body.[19] These results are amazing. If you can't do that -- if you can't do 9 minutes of exercise per week, you might as well just hang it up now because there's really not much hope for a healthy future.

If you'd like more information on the PACE program, I would strongly recommend purchasing Dr. Al Sears' book, Rediscover Your Native Fitness.

STRENGTH TRAINING

We need to do strength training. It doesn't have to be anything major. You don't have to go to the gym and bench 350 pounds for 10 repetitions. But we need to do something to send that signal to our body to build more muscle mass. This does not require a gym, if you have a floor (most people do), you can do push-ups, you can do sit-ups. One of my favorite pieces of exercise equipment is called a "power stand"—a frame that stands about 7 feet tall. It allows one to do chin-ups, pull-ups, dips, push-ups and more. With strength training, there are diminishing returns with each set that we do. I realize the idea of doing 2 or 3 reps has been promoted for a long time, but there are diminishing returns with that second and third rep, compared to the gains of that first rep. The whole idea with that first rep, however, is to do whatever you until you are fatigued. If you are lifting weights and you are doing 30 repetitions, it is not enough weight. I don't care whether you're 10 or 110 years old, these same concepts need to be applied. That means if you are doing more than 10 reps comfortably, it is not enough weight, or you need to modify whatever exercise it is that you are doing. If you're doing push-ups, go deeper. Get a set of Perfect Push-ups or those push-up bars that allow you to do deeper push-ups. You can take them slower through the entire range of motion. If you can do more than 10, it's not enough weight. You need to increase the weight until you are only able to do 8 to10 repetitions to fatigue -- and at the end of those 8-10 repetitions, you should feel wiped out. For most of us, strength training three times per week is going to be enough to maintain the strength that we need.

BAHADORI LEANNESS PROGRAM

One last aspect of exercise that has an impact on neuroprotection is a concept called the Bahadori leanness program. The Bahadori leanness principle uses planned "mini-fasts" to manage body fat. In general, it is not acceptable to skip meals. However, when the meal is skipped, in its place is substituted a relatively high-level aerobic activity. Specific supplements are used to facilitate the efficient use of calories to burn fat and maintain muscle. So basically, what you're doing is skipping the meal, but instead of sitting at a desk reading emails, you're actually undergoing a high-level aerobic activity.[20]

So how does this affect the brain? From an evolutionary standpoint, imagine you were hungry and hadn't eaten in a while. You were on the hunt and were getting closer to your prey. That is a very important time for us to have a strong neurologic focus. The last thing you want to occur if you hadn't eaten for days and were hunting prey is this: Straight ahead of you, you see the prey in the brush. So you jump up to chase it down and lose neurologic clarity, have a seizure and pass out – or, worse, lapse into a coma. That would be the worst time, and it does not contribute to long-term survival.

Because of that, the Bahadori leanness principle makes sense because it coincides with what we are designed for when viewed from an evolutionary standpoint. It must be said that anyone adopting this program must follow the specifically outlined principles. Haphazard skipping of meals, insufficient exercising or lack of specific nutrients may very well lead to weight gains and to less than ideal brain health. Dr. Babak Bahadori has published a book with the specifics to his program, which also includes additional steps for healthy living that go beyond exercise.

CHAPTER SIX SUMMARY AND ACTION STEPS

Summary:

1. Exercise is NOT an option; it is required for a healthy brain.

2. Continual aerobic exercise is not as effective as interval-type exercise.
3. The PACE program seems to fit well with the way our bodies are designed.
4. Strength training needs to be a portion of your workout routine.
5. The Bahadori Leanness program combines weight loss with brain protection.

Action Steps:

1. If you are not exercising, figure out what form of aerobic activity fits into your lifestyle. This can be walking, running, jump-roping, elliptical or hiking.
2. For weight / strength-training, keep it simple. Target the larger muscle groups such as the hamstrings, quadriceps, gluts, abdominals, chest muscles, biceps and triceps. Personally, I feel that chin-ups, pull-ups, push-ups, sit-ups and dips fill the need of my muscle building activities. This group of exercises requires no gym membership. Sit-ups and push-ups can be done if you have a floor, which most of us probably have.
3. If the Bahardi Leanness Program appeals to you, look in the resource section for contact information.

In Chapter 7, we will look at some specific dietary approaches that have been shown to have powerful effects on controlling both seizures and migraines.

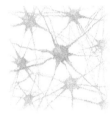

Chapter 7

DIET

We have already discussed the low-calorie, high-phytonutrient approach to the way we should all be eating to protect our brains. Here we will outline some additional tools to augment this dietary pattern. Specifically, it is the elimination and the ketogenic diet.

ELIMINATION DIET

Food allergies can play a role in how healthy your brain is. There have been multiple studies looking at the ability of food sensitivities and the elimination diet to reduce the frequency, and some cases eliminate, both seizures and migraines.[21,22,23,24]

Many times patients come in and note that they have been checked for food allergies. They went to an allergist and had a skin scratch test performed. The skin scratch test works for the immediate onset, known as IgE, type of allergies. I consider and I call them a hard-wired allergy. For the test, the skin is scratched with an allergen and, if you have a reaction to that antigen (such as pollen, mites, peanuts), you will develop a wheal over the scratch as early as in a couple of hours, or as long as a couple of days.

Traditionally though, when we're talking about food allergies, we're really looking at sensitivities – things that our bodies had become sensitive to, based on the environment we are in or the high level of exposure we have to some types of food. These are referred to as delayed-type hypersensitivities, or IgG4. While the blood can be checked for these types of reactions, this approach is far from ideal because it has the potential to miss things we are sensitive to.

High on the list of foods we may be sensitive to is dairy. Arguably the greatest marketing success in history has brainwashed us into thinking that dairy is a good thing and builds strong minds, bones and muscles. However, when you really start to look at the research on dairy, it is something that we should be avoiding. You'll find that most physicians who practice functional medicine and who understand more about nutrition are no fans of dairy.

An elimination diet involves at least two weeks of avoiding common allergens. High on the list of common allergens are dairy, wheat, corn and soy. However, there are others that may be affecting your brain and producing headaches and/or seizures. The idea with doing a two-week elimination diet is sometimes it takes the body a while to respond to what it is exposed to.

There was a study several years ago where it was determined that dairy in a group of children was causing constipation. When they pulled the kids off dairy foods, the constipation went away. When they reintroduced a single, isolated serving of dairy after a period of their being dairy-free, some children took up to 10 days for the constipation to show up from one single exposure.

I don't know about you, but I don't remember what I had to eat yesterday for lunch, let alone 10 days ago. Hence, the two-week elimination diet gives our bodies a chance to get rid of all of those backlogged responses from the food that we've eaten in the prior two weeks.

At the end of the elimination diet, foods are reintroduced one at a time for a single exposure. So, you've gone two weeks. You're starting to feel better. You haven't had any headaches. You try dairy. You just have a single glass, or a couple of sips, and if your headache comes back in the next couple of days, then you know dairy is off the list, at least for a long enough time period until your body's sensitivity to it is reduced. You then repat that with the other allergens – again, reintroducing them at one point in time and evaluating for a response.

The elimination diet works very well in those people who have frequent symptoms. If you have a migraine every two or three months, the problem is you have to do the elimination diet for that period of time to determine if that food sensitivity is playing a role. You would do the food challenge at this point.

There are multiple resources for the specifics on an elimination diet on the Internet if you choose to go that direction. If this seems like it may be difficult, remember that an elimination diet is almost a necessary tool to determine which foods your body may be sensitive to.

KETOGENIC DIET

The ketogenic diet is probably one of the more powerful tools to manage epilepsy. Interesting enough, it was used almost exclusively for seizures up until the 1920s and fell out of favor when drug companies started to develop anti-epileptic drugs. Fast forward 90 years, and now the ketogenic diet is only recommended for children who have had intractable seizures that are not controlled by medication. It seems backwards that the diet is put at the tail end, rather than the front end, of treatment.[25]

Despite strong research supporting the use of the ketogenic diet, few neurologists recommend this approach. Consistently across studies, a third of the children on the ketogenic diet have greater than 90% seizure reduction. A third have more than 50% seizure reduction. This outcome is stronger than any medications available. We're talking about a pretty powerful therapeutic approach.

There are a few variations of the diet. Many have become familiar with the ketogenic diet because it is similar to the approach taken during the Atkins diet used for weight loss. For weight loss, the ketogenic diet has some serious shortcomings, so the risk-versus-benefit ratio does not favor the benefits, especially when many other options for healthy weight loss are available. However, you can modify the ketogenic diet or the Atkins diet from the traditional diet to better fit your lifestyle. There are resources at the end of this book where you can learn much more about the ketogenic diet and how to adapt it to your life, if that is a direction you choose to take.

The original ketogenic diet had 4:1 fat-to-carbohydrate ratio. The problem is these restrictions can be hard to follow long term, and if too many carbohydrates are eaten, seizures can return almost instantly. Another problem with the ketogenic diet is the lack of soluble fiber, increasing the risk of constipation. However, that is very easy to fix with 400 milligrams of magnesium before bedtime and probiotics. As an added bonus, the supplementation with magnesium is good for the brain and is very important for mitochondrial function. Thus, there are a variety of ways to affect the constipation and make that a non-issue.

The modified Atkins diet has a 1:1 ratio of fats to carbohydrates. Recent studies show that this was just as effective and much more tolerable in the long run for those patients who were taking it. Because of that, the modified Atkins diet may be a great tool to start implementing. And, as mentioned, this dietary approach, is not done as a single therapy. This should be done in conjunction with everything else noted in managing the seizures – the supplementation, the exercise and the stress management. Diet is not a single, isolated therapy to be used.

Another variation of the ketogenic diet is the polyunsaturated ketogenic diet. That is probably not only one of the more palatable, but also one of the best to use long term.

In the polyunsaturated ketogenic diet, the type of fat intake is principally polyunsaturated fat, such as those found in nuts, seeds and fish. In general, polyunsaturated fats are a liquid at room temperature. We can modify fats like peanut oil, which is naturally a liquid at room temperature, by hydrogenating them to make them a solid at room temperature. But in dong that, the health benefits of the oils become damaging effects. These are NOT what we're talking about in the polyunsaturated ketogenic diet.

The polyunsaturated ketogenic diet is much higher in omega-3 fatty acid content, which is a strong positive for our brains. We cover that later. So obviously a diet that takes in much higher amounts of omega-3 fatty acids is going to be very good for your brain. Although the research is not quite certain yet as to why the ketogenic diet works, many researchers believe these polyunsaturated fats play the most significant role. Future research will hopefully elucidate the mechanisms by which the ketogenic diet protects the brain.

GLUTEN-FREE DIET

In the past few years, there has been much increased awareness of the problems associated with the allergy to wheat referred to as Celiac Disease, or gluten sensitivity. Whatever you call it, it is here to stay. But exactly how far do

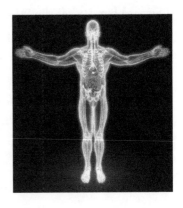

the negative health effects of celiac disease run? And can this affect the brain?

Let's start with the basics. Traditionally, celiac disease was a condition where an allergy to a protein called gluten in certain grains (most commonly wheat, barley and rye, but also in trace amounts in oats) set up a reaction where the immune system begins to destroy itself called an auto-immune reaction. This reaction destroys the pockets of tissue lining the gut called the villa. The total surface area of the small intestine is usually estimated to be close to that of a tennis court. This is because all of the villi lining the intestinal tract increase the surface area. Now, consider this tennis court shrinking to the size of a ping pong table. Nutrient malabsorption will result along with a long list of other bad things.

That was then, but this is now...

Over time, we have come to understand that the scenario of celiac disease described above is the far end of a spectrum that starts with only a mild sensitivity that can be picked up via stool sampling at specific labs like www.enterolab.com. The problem is that the inflammation set up by exposure to a common allergen such as gluten wreaks subtle havoc that compounds over the course of years and decades. That can lead to conditions like Type 1 diabetes, thyroid problems and bone problems. But can something occurring in the gut actually affect something as far away as the brain?

The answer is a clear yes. Almost 20 years ago, researchers were calling for evaluation of gluten sensitivity in any undiagnosed neurological disorder[26]. New research has begun to demonstrate very strong links between epilepsy and celiac disease[27].

Researchers found that, those with the far spectrum of celiac disease (those with the destruction of the villi noted under a microscope) had a 40% increased risk of developing epilepsy.

Two very important thoughts come to mind.

First, this study looked at the far spectrum of celiac disease, showing a 40% increase. But what about the rest of the spectrum of those who react to gluten? What if we looked in reverse to see how many epileptics had sensitivity to gluten? We may be surprised at what we would find.

Secondly, we have already covered the ketogenic diet. As mentioned, researchers are not really sure how the diet works to control seizures, although speculation about the type of fat being eaten is key. But, on the ketogenic diet, most grains are eliminated or severely reduced. Could gluten really be the key to the success of the ketogenic diet? Based on current research, it may very well be the answer researchers have been looking for.

CHAPTER SEVEN SUMMARY AND ACTION STEPS

Summary:

1. For migraines, food sensitivities can play a very large role in causing headaches.
2. Dairy, wheat, corn and soy are very common allergens.
3. Blood tests for IgG4 sensitivies are available, but not as good as an elimination diet.

4. An elimination diet eliminates a list of common allergens for two weeks. Foods are then reintroduced, one at a time, to check to see if this food creates a headache.

5. The ketogenic diet is a diet that is low in carbohydrate intake.

6. The ketogenic diet has been shown to be far more powerful at controlling seizures than medications.

7. Because of the perceived difficulties with long-term use of the ketogenic diet, variations of the ketogenic diet have been tried: standard diet is 4:1 fat: carbs, modified 1:1 ratio, polyunsaturated ketogenic diet.

8. Gluten is a protein contained in certain grains like wheat, barley and rye. In susceptible individuals, gluten causes the body to attack itself. As a result, neurological damage can occur, which may be linked to seizures.

Action Steps:

1. For migraines, use the elimination diet to identify foods that trigger your headaches. Visit the resource section to find out more information on an elimination diet.

2. In epilepsy, if your seizures are not controlled by medications (intractable epilepsy) then discuss the use of the ketogenic diet with your neurologists. If they are not supportive, find a new one.

3. If you decide the ketogenic diet is an approach that you would like to try, decide which of the types of

ketogenic diet will work for you (standard, modified, polyunsaturated). I personally am most supportive of the polyunsaturated version. Visit the resources section for more information.

4. Consider a gluten-free diet for four weeks and evaluate how you feel. In today's marketplace, the availability of gluten-free foods has exploded, making this a much easier lifestyle to lead.

In Chapter 8, we will begin to examine supplements that have been shown to improve brain function. Even the addition of simple supplements can have strong, positive effects on migraine headaches and seizures

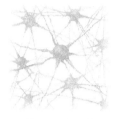

Chapter 8

SUPPLEMENTS

Supplements absolutely play a role in protecting our brain. My viewpoint on supplements is nothing replaces a good, quality, healthy lifestyle. Supplements should act as an insurance policy in case you don't happen to get everything that you need or in case your stress levels have exceeded what your body can protect against at that given time. So the idea of supplements is not to replace a good, quality lifestyle. We need to make sure that is important right upfront.

ESSENTIAL FATTY ACIDS

The supplements designed to protect the brain come in a couple of different categories. One of the most important categories is essential fatty acids, such as your "fish oil-type" supplement. Essential fatty acids are called "essential" because our bodies cannot manufacture them so we have to consume them in our diet. Generally, the ones that have been shown to be most protective for humans are the omega-3 fatty acids, alpha-linolenic acid (ALA), docosahexaenoic acid (DHA), and eicosapentaenoic acid (EPA). Ideally, we should obtain these fats from our diets.

Principal sources of ALA are mainly plant-based, such as flaxseeds, walnuts, chia seeds and grains like salba. Generally, we don't think of ALA as being as protective to the brain as DHA. However, some studies have indicated that ALA may have a potent ability to protect the brain against the oxidative stress induced by a seizure in animals.[28] In addition to protecting the brain, ALA also has well-documented benefits on the heart and reductions in the risk of prostate cancer for men. Overall, however, we should not think of ALA as the principal fatty acid protecting the brain.

EPA and DHA are generally what we consider "fish oil." Herbivore fish get these fatty acids from the algae and seaweed that they eat. That's one of the principal sources of DHA. Certain herbivore fish will eat the DHA in the plants leading to concentrated levels of DHA in the fish. Bigger fish subsequently eat these fish, and the fish oil content continues to increase. That is the pathway of DHA from plants to fish. That's also why farm-raised fish is not a good alternative to wild-caught fish for consumption. Farm-raised fish are fed a meal based on corn, which does not have the same healthy fats from the algae and seaweed that the wild herbivore fish like tilapia, salmon and cod eat.

Fish oil supplements come into play here. Generally, we'll push people towards the EPA and DHA and focus lastly on the ALA. As far as levels go, in general, higher is better. We don't see too many side-effects of higher levels of fish oil unless somebody happens to be on blood thinners, like Coumadin or Plavix. But in this case, the patient is usually monitored at a clinic, and increased intake of omega-3 fatty acids should be taken into account. If you are on blood thinners and would like to increase your intake of fish oil supplements, this goal should be discussed with the clinic so that the doctors there are well aware of any changes.

As mentioned, higher levels of essential fatty-acid supplementation are generally better. Keep in mind that a typical fish oil capsule is about one gram. That's not just fish oil. The capsules usually contain glycerin as well. It depends on the potency of the fish oil or potency of the capsule. A typical capsule may have 300 milligrams to as high as 744 milligrams of omega-3-fatty acids. Keep in mind that most bottle labels give the dosages in milligrams, so if you want to take three grams of fish oil per day, that will require much more than three capsules to get to those levels depending on the potency in that particular fish-oil capsule.

I recommend splitting up the doses of fish oil. In general, with the higher quality fish oils repeating (burping up that wonderful fish smell) is not much of an issue because there are fewer contaminants and a lower likelihood of fat to be rancid inside the capsule. By splitting the dosages, repeating is less likely to occur. Taking them with meals will also help increase the absorption as the digestive processes rev up to absorb the other oils and fats in the food that was eaten.

ANTIOXIDANT SUPPLEMENTS

The other class of supplements that can aid in protecting the brain are the antioxidants.[29,30] Interestingly, some of the more commonly used medications to treat seizures, such as zonisamide, may derive some of their benefit by acting as an antioxidant.[29] Antioxidants carry names such as coenzyme Q10, alpha-lipoic acid, Vitamin E, Vitamin C and greens-type drinks. These are just some of the many that are found in a typical nutrition or supplement store. A few of the more commons ones will be covered here.

COENZYME Q10 (COQ10)

Top of the list is coenzyme Q10 or CoQ10. The other term for CoQ10 is ubiquinone, meaning that it is ubiquitous – it is present in all of our cells. Its presence is absolutely essential for our cells to make energy. We've already talked about the smoke from the free radicals in the process of generating ATP. Coenzyme Q10 is absolutely essential in the process of generating ATP as well as protecting against free radicals. So taking it from the supplement standpoint can help protect the brain and the neurons as they start to produce more and more ATP and the subsequent free radicals. Coenzyme Q10 can quench those free radicals. Research supports the use of CoQ10 as an adjunctive (add-on) therapy along with anti-epileptic medications such as Lamictal.[32]

From a dosage standpoint, again, in general more is better. However, CoQ10 is an expensive supplement. Generally, 100 to 400 mgs per day fit into most people's budgets. However, it has been shown in clinical studies to be effective in doses of up to 1,200 to 2,000 mgs per day. But then we're talking about $200 to $300 a month in CoQ10 cost. So it gets a little prohibitive for most people.

ALPHA-LIPOIC ACID

Alpha-lipoic acid (ALA) packs quite a punch. Studies backed by the National Institutes of Health, dating as far back as the mid-1970s, demonstrated strong improvement in patients with liver failure and were on liver transplant lists. They were given 400 milligrams of ALA per day. ALA has the same potential to protect the brain at dosages typically around 400 milligrams per day.

VITAMIN E

Next one on the list is vitamin E. There has been quite a bit of controversy surrounding vitamin E's over the years in wake of a study demonstrating that those people taking vitamin E actually had a slightly increased risk of heart problems. As a result, many doctors who don't understand vitamin E started to tell patients to avoid or stop taking vitamin E.

The reality is that vitamin E actually comes in about eight different forms. They fall into the tocotrienols and tocopherols. I call them cousins of one another. Most of what people think of when they think of and take vitamin E is the alpha-tocopherol acid form. Interestingly, when you look at the history of vitamin E, you find it is not the most potent vitamin E that nature makes. It is not the most protective for the heart or the brain. It is merely through an odd series of events that the alpha tocopherol gained ascendancy as the dominant supplement.

Mother Nature actually produces much higher levels of gamma tocopherol. The problem is when you get high levels of alpha, we actually see a drop in the blood levels of the gamma tocopherol. Given that the gamma tocopherol is so protective to the heart, we could easily see a problem of giving too much alpha-tocopherol as a supplement (which is the principal form in supplements). This would lower the levels of gamma and create potential problems with the heart. Not following this recommendation has led to misinformation and confusion recently as several studies found a small increase in heart-disease risk in those taking vitamin E. So cardiologists, unfamiliar with all of the forms of vitamin E, began to tell their patients to stop taking it. What they did not realize is that the gamma tocopherol has the strongest ability to protect the heart. BUT, giving too much of one type of vitamin E, in this case the alpha form, actually LOWERED the levels of the protective gamma form! Of course we didn't see any protection to the heart!! It's a perfect example of how we need to produce balance when it comes to antioxidant protection for our bodies.

The take home message with vitamin E is to take a broad spectrum vitamin E supplement that contains a blend of tocopherols and tocotrienols, just like nature. Most health food stores carry these better quality vitamin E supplements.

The recommended range is anywhere from 200 to 400 IUs of tocopherols per day.

VITAMIN C

Next on our list is vitamin C. I recommend taking vitamin C and vitamin E together due to their synergistic effect. Vitamin E is a fat-soluble antioxidant and vitamin C is water-soluble. We talked earlier (see page 29) about how vitamin E can actually become a pro-oxidant if it doesn't have a corresponding water-soluble antioxidant to work with. So vitamin C and vitamin E work well together as a team. A dosage of 1,000 to 2,000 mg of vitamin C daily is a good place to start.

MELATONIN

Melatonin is a hormone produced deep in the brain in a gland called the pineal gland. It has traditionally been thought of as the hormone that helps to regulate our sleep/wake cycle. Sunlight hitting the retina halts the pineal gland's production of melatonin. As the sun goes down and it gets darker, melatonin levels rise because they are no longer being inhibited.

Recently, however, there has been a growing understanding of the ability of melatonin to act as a potent antioxidant within the brain, either directly or through the increase in production of our brain's own antioxidant systems.[33] This is why proper sleep patterns may be critical to the brain, as they ensure that melatonin levels are optimal when they are supposed to be elevated. Shift workers and insomniacs may be particularly vulnerable.

Melatonin has also been shown to have anti-seizure activities in animal studies.[34,35] Because of promising results in research studies, its low cost and its excellent safety profile, researchers are beginning to suggest the use of melatonin in the treatment of epilepsy.[36] Melatonin levels are found to be low in chronic migraine sufferers as well, and, for this reason, melatonin has also been considered as a potential therapeutic supplement for migraine headaches as well.[37]

From a supplementation standpoint, melatonin is a very inexpensive supplement. I always recommend starting at a .5 mg dose because higher doses may cause nightmares and grogginess the next morning. I have patients progress slowly up from there, rarely exceeding a 3 mg dose.

MULTIVITAMIN

Another important addition is a good quality multivitamin. It covers the bases on so many grounds, making sure that you can obtain a broad spectrum of vitamins and minerals. To qualify a good quality multivitamin, I always rule out the "one-per-day" type of multivitamins. How many times do we need to eat a meal per day? Can we have just one meal in the morning and that'll be enough for the rest of the day? Of course the answer is no, so this should be no different with our multivitamins.

In a "one-per-day" multivitamin, the water-soluble vitamins in the formulation that are taken in the morning will not be stored by the body. This leaves you without these same water-soluble vitamins in the afternoon or evening if you need them, such as under times of increase physical or emotional stress. So the better quality multivitamins will have serving sizes anywhere from three to six per day. I recommend patients break the servings up between two or three meals during the day, such as with breakfast and dinner. There's a variety of other things you need to look at on the label to make sure it's a good quality multivitamins, but ruling out the "one-per-day" multivitamins knocks out the vast majority of the lower quality vitamins on the market.

VINPOCETINE

Vinpocetine is a compound present in the periwinkle plant and has been used for many years to support memory and overall brain function. While there have been no human studies on vinpocetine's effect on seizures or migraines, the animal research studies being done are well worth a mention. This compound has the ability to prevent glutamate release in hippocampal tissue from the brain that is far superior to many anti-seizure medications. While the anti-seizure medications carbamazepine, phenytoin, lamotrigine and oxcarbazepine were able to lower the release of glutamate by 50-60%, vinpocetine was able to completely shut it down, and at lower doses. Pretty impressive. Topimarate was not able to affect glutamate release at all.

Because research into natural compounds has a tendency to run very slow, it may be years or even decades before we see greater research on vinpocetine. If the results of current studies are any indication of the results of future studies, this compound may end up as one of the more powerful anti-seizure supplements available.[38]

VITAMIN B6

Also known by the much more important sounding name "pyroxidine," vitamin B6 plays an integral role in healthy neurotransmitter function, specifically as it relates to glutamate and GABA. The enzyme glutamic acid decarboxylase uses vitamin B6 to convert glutamate to GABA. This means that, without enough B6, glutamate, the excitatory /proseizure neurotransmitter, may be elevated at the same time that GABA, the inhibitory and protective neurotransmitter, is low. Not a good combination for the brain.

B6 needs to be activated in the liver to become pyroxidine-5-phosphate (P5P), which is the active form the body uses. While the recommended daily allowance (RDA) hovers around 1.3 mg per day, therapeutic doses frequently fall in the 100-200 mg per-day range. While it is possible to develop a reversible nerve problem with overdose of B6, this is not commonly seen in dosages below 500 mg per day and is reversible once the B6 is stopped.

VITAMIN D

Next and probably one of the more important supplements is vitamin D, also known as the "sunshine vitamin." We live in a society that has promoted the idea of slapping on SPF 80 just to walk to the car, and we're now paying a price for that. There are many studies that have found associations between low levels of vitamin D and a variety of conditions. Most notably is osteoporosis but many types of cancer, heart disease, high blood pressure and depression are also on the list.

Vitamin D is also known to act as an anti-convulsant. This is important to remember because a lot of the anti-epileptic drugs – the AEDs – actually lower levels of vitamin D in the blood. So, we have a compound that actually helps protect the brain, but the drugs that we use to control seizures actually lower the levels of a substance that can protect the brain. This creates somewhat of a conundrum. This may also be the reason why most AEDs also have a negative effect on bone density, again strongly supporting the use of vitamin D in migraines and epilepsy.

Taking vitamin D as a supplement is very inexpensive and the safety margins on the dosages of Vitamin D are quite wide (toxicity with vitamin D is not noted until the blood levels are over 200 nmol/L, which is a pretty difficult level to reach). However, if someone has any concerns about taking higher dosages of Vitamin D, blood levels can easily be checked. Optimal blood levels are between 60 and 100 nmol/L, although most labs will consider 20 and higher as normal.

There are times when vitamin D supplementation may be of concern. One such situation is with the use of thiazide diuretics that raise the level of calcium (due to reduced excretion).[39] Also patients with the auto-immune granulomatous disorder sarcoidosis need to be a little bit more cautious. Other conditions known to increase the levels of calcium in the blood like histoplasmosis or hyperparathyroidism require care with supplementation. If someone has any questions or concerns, they should obviously discuss them with their primary care doctor. In addition, there are a lot of great resources on the Internet.

Recommended dosages depend on several factors, such as how much sun exposure you get or at what latitude you live. (Higher latitudes get less direct sunlight so our bodies make less vitamin D. Near the equator, vitamin D production is at its highest). Many mistakenly believe that they get enough sun exposure and that supplementation is not needed. However, there is concern that the sun passing through glass allows only UVA penetration, actually breaking down the production of vitamin D in the skin. So if you drive around all summer with the windows up in your car and the AC cranked, you may actually be lowering your vitamin D levels. Furthermore, it takes at least 8 hours to fully produce and absorb the vitamin D our skin is trying to produce, so showering at night may lower blood vitamin D levels.[40] There is also concern of particulate matter in the atmosphere blocking UVB penetration and also lowering vitamin D levels.

Because of these concerns, I generally start patients anywhere from 2,000 to 4,000 IU per day, although it is sometimes higher, depending upon the clinical scenario. Having your bone density checked can further help determine vitamin D need. In our clinic, we strongly recommend patients have their first bone density testing in their 20s and 30s so they aren't waiting until they're 55 or 60 and are now at the crisis stage for treating low-bone density.

For supplementation, liquid forms are going to be much cheaper and easier to use. Vitamin D can actually be dosed on a weekly basis. The vitamin D we use in the office has 2,000 IUs per drop; if someone is on 2,000 IUs per day, they can actually do seven drops once a week. It is one of the easiest and cheapest supplements to take.

CHAPTER EIGHT SUMMARY AND ACTION STEPS

Summary:

1. Supplements can play a strong role in keeping your brain healthy.

2. Fish oils (EPA/DHA) help to stabilize the cell well of our neurons and improve the way our cells communicate. The healthier the cell wall, the better that cell is able to control when it fires and when it should not fire.

3. Antioxidants like CoQ10, alpha lipoic acid, vitamin E, vitamin C and greens-type drinks can provide ammo for our neurons to protect against oxidative stress and subsequent damage to their internal machinery.

4. Melatonin is a hormone produced deep in the brain that can help regulate our sleep/wake cycle. It also functions as a strong antioxidant within the brain and has been shown to help lower seizure rates in animals.

5. A good quality multivitamin is very important to give a strong foundation of vitamins and minerals. A good quality multivitamin does not include the popular brands that are taken once per day.

6. The compound vinpocetine, derived from the periwinkle plant, has shown some very powerful

anti-seizure properties in animal studies. While the research is still in its early stages, it is a supplement that may become a strong player as more research accumulates.

7. Vitamin B6 is essential to help convert glutamate, which excites the brain, to GABA, which calms the brain.

8. Vitamin D is a hormone that is deficient in a very large percentage of the population, even in sun-drenched areas. It plays an important role in brain health and is even known to have some anti-seizure properties. Many drugs that are used to treat migraines and seizures will lower levels of vitamin D. This will lower the ability of vitamin D to protect the brain and is likely a reason why many drugs for migraines and seizures are bad for the bones. Basically, vitamin D supplementation is required if you are reading this.

Action Steps:

1. Fish oil supplement at 3 grams. This is 3,000 mg of the actual omega-3-fatty acids, so you'll have to look at the bottle label and do the math.

2. Daily supplementation levels: CoQ10 (100-400 mg-basically as much as you can afford), alpha lipoic acid (400 mg), a mixed tocopherol vitamin E (200 mg), vitamin C (2,000 mg), greens-type drink.

3. If sleep is a problem, add melatonin starting at .5 mg/day about one hour before desired bedtime.

4. Vitamin B6 (pyroxidine) at 100-200 mg/day.
5. Vitamin D supplementation at 2,000-4,000 IU/day. Higher levels are usually recommended but should be followed with blood work to make sure levels don't go too high (although that is rare).

In Chapter 9, we will look at how our sense of smell can actually increase or lower our risk of seizures and headaches and some recommendations of the scents that have been shown in the research to have a positive impact on brain function

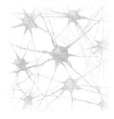

Chapter 9   **AROMATHERAPY**

nother tool that can be brought into play to help the brain is aromatherapy. It may initially sound strange that something as simple as a scent can actually help to control seizures. However, there is actually quite a bit of research surrounding the old wives' tale that the "shoe" smell can control seizures. This may have been what actually prompted studies on the ability of aromatherapy to calm the brain.

On the flip side, many migraine sufferers will find that certain scents can trigger a headache. This can include such compounds as perfumes or cleaning agents. These patients can usually list the smells that they know will kick off a headache.

There are studies where aromatherapy has been shown to increase GABA levels. Remember that GABA is one of the more potent neurotransmitters and calms and soothes the brain. Lavender and clary sage are probably two of the most commonly essential oils found in the medical literature.[41,42]

As a nice simple tool with very little cost, it is something else that can be used to help calm down your brain.

CHAPTER NINE SUMMARY AND ACTION STEPS

Summary:

1. Smells can positively and negatively impact brain health.
2. Aromatherapy has been shown to increase GABA levels in the brain. Clary sage and lavender are two of the most commonly researched essential oils.

Action Steps:

1. Any oils that are used should be essential oils. Lower quality oils that contain perfumes can actually trigger headaches. Look in the resource section for some companies that you can order very high quality oils from.

In Chapter 10, we will begin to look at the contribution that hormones make to brain health and our risk of migraines and seizures. We will help identify methods by which you can improve your own hormone levels so that you can achieve long-term brain health

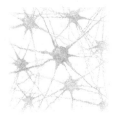

HORMONES

N o discussion on brain health would be complete without the topic of hormones. Obviously, every hormone plays a role. Some, like cortisol, insulin, epinephrine, estrogen, testosterone, and progesterone are larger players than others. Conversely, our overall state of health has an effect on hormone levels.

MENSTRUAL MIGRAINES

Before we begin talking about the specific hormones, we need to address menstrual migraines. There can actually be a very easy fix to many menstrual migraines. We've already discussed oxidative stress, and one of the factors that plays a role in oxidative stress is the ability to carry oxygen to our brains. If the

75

brain doesn't have enough oxygen, our mitochondria won't be able to produce the ATP that we need, and the brain is not able to stop firing when it's not supposed to fire. So, any drop in the ability to deliver oxygen to the brain can create problems. This is exactly the state that many women experience in the second half of their menstrual cycles as the lining of the endometrium begins to build, removing red blood cells from circulation and reducing the ability of the blood to bring oxygen to the brain. That can be a very subtle drop in red blood cell level, but given how sensitive the brain is to changes in oxygen levels, that can be enough to trigger a migraine in already sensitive people.

Through the years, I've had patients who have suffered with menstrual migraines. The migraine starts on the first day of the menstrual cycle, or just before. In those cases, it is always worth an attempt at adding 10-15 milligrams of a higher quality (i.e. citrate, gluconate) iron supplement starting from day 14 (the beginning of ovulation) through the next 7 to 14 days. This can be just enough to continue to support the ability of the remaining red blood cells to deliver the much-needed oxygen to the brain cells It doesn't work for everybody, but if it works, it's a very simple fix for menstrual migraine sufferers.

PROGESTERONE AND ALLOPREGNONALONE

Probably one of the most important players when it comes to protecting the brain is the hormone progesterone. In premenopausal women, progesterone comes mainly from both the adrenal glands as well as from the healthy release of the ovum at the time of ovulation. In postmenopausal women, the source of progesterone is primarily the adrenal glands.

Obviously if a woman becomes pregnant, then the highest source of progesterone comes from the placenta. A pregnant woman's progesterone levels can be 10 times higher than a non-pregnant woman.

As a side note, progesterone may also play a strong role in seizures and in migraines that occur in males as well. However, without a menstrual cycle that accompanies changes in hormone levels, it is difficult to correlate symptoms with changes in progesterone production in men.

So, what's so important about progesterone? Progesterone actually gets converted to a neurosteroid called allopregnanolone. A neurosteroid is a hormone that affects the way a brain cell functions. This compound acts on GABA receptors. GABA stands for gamma-aminobutyric acid. When GABA lands on the receptor site of a neuron, it puts the brakes on the neurological system. It has a strong, sedative, calming effect on the brain. Drugs that affect these pathways, like valium, have been used to control seizures for decades. Allopregnanolone is thought to be the most potent anti-seizure compound on the planet – synthetic or natural.

So we start to see that progesterone has a massive impact on how well the brain is functioning and our ability to have or not have seizures. One of the premier researchers along this path is Dr. Andrew Herzog out of the neuroendocrinology unit at Harvard University. His group has published several clinical trials on progesterone for temporal lobe epilepsy with very good results.[43]

Given the importance of progesterone in this process, we need to make sure that women are secreting optimal levels of progesterone and allowing for the best chance for conversion to allopregnanolone. Allopregnanolone is actually a very strong target right now for several pharmaceutical researchers aiming to come up with a synthetic version. Once they do, this drug will probably launch itself to the head of the list for preferred anti-seizure medications.

As an FYI, women who experience seizures in the later portion of the luteal phase of their menstrual cycle (day 14-28), this type of seizure is referred to a catamenial seizures, or seizures related to their menstrual cycle. This type of seizure is strongly associated with rapid drops in progesterone levels.

To optimize the production of progesterone, we want to make sure that the ovaries and the adrenal glands are functioning properly. Many are not aware that a large production of progesterone actually comes from the adrenal cortex. So, if we've got too much stress or are chronically stressed, we may not be producing the progesterone that we need and increase our risk for seizures or migraines.

The reduced progesterone as a result of chronic stress has to do with the reserve of the adrenal glands. They can only produce so much "stuff," and when we are stressed, these reserves are shunted over to the production of higher levels of cortisol. This leaves less "stuff" to make the other two hormones, aldosterone and dehydroepiandrosterone (DHEA). Since the body uses DHEA to produce progesterone, this means that stress will lower our production of progesterone. I cannot reiterate too often that stress reduction becomes a major player in improving the health of your brain.

INSULIN RESISTANCE, PREDIABETES AND PROGESTERONE

In today's society, another important factor in reducing the amount of progesterone in pre-menopausal women is that, in the pre-diabetic state, the high levels of the hormone insulin dramatically affect the way the ovaries function. The pre-diabetic state is arguably one of the most dangerous states for the human body. It greatly increases the risk for almost every single chronic disease. Pre-diabetes is one of the greatest problems that I see in patients every single day.

Everyone understands that diabetes is not good for us. However, many physicians and their patients are unaware of just how dangerous it is to be pre-diabetic. This is the analogy I use for those who are pre-diabetic. I have patients who come in my office and, based on a number of factors they have, such as blood work, increased weight around the middle or high blood pressure, I discuss with them that they might be pre-diabetic. The standard patient reply is, "Well, my doctor checked that, and he said I'm not diabetic." You can almost see the audible "Whew."

This is because most of us are under the impression that if we're not diabetic, we're okay. But in reality, this is the equivalent of a cigarette smoker saying, "You know what, my doctor checked me for lung cancer, and he said I'm okay, so I'm just going to keep smoking." Pre-diabetes is arguably just as dangerous for us, and possibly even more so, than smoking.

One thing that goes along with being pre-diabetic is the elevated levels of insulin flowing around in our bloodstreams. When that happens, we have a problem with the body converting testosterone to estrogen, causing testosterone levels to increase. Testosterone then starts to mess with the ovaries' ability to produce progesterone. That's why, with polycystic ovary syndrome, which is one of the most common causes of infertility in women, we get a lot of androgynous (male hormone) type features like acne or facial hair, because of the elevated testosterone.

In the above scenario, in a pre-menopausal female, when the ovary releases the ovum at ovulation, the testosterone keeps this newly released egg from fully functioning. This leads to a drop in the amount of progesterone produced and therefore less of it circulating in the bloodstream. With reduced circulating progesterone, there is less conversion to allopregnonalone in the brain and a reduced ability to calm down the brain. You've lost one of the more potent hormones that protect the brain.

Hopefully you are beginning to see that protecting our brain is truly a comprehensive approach and needs to be viewed from all angles. You are not going to be able to take this or that drug or this supplement or just exercise and it's all going to better.

STRESS HORMONES

Now we move onto the stress hormones. Acute stress is actually very good for the brain. If you think about it, this makes a lot of sense. If we had a saber-toothed tiger jump out of the underbrush looking to attack us, the last thing we'd want is for our brain to get all fuzzy. Instead, acute stress snaps our brain, and our neurons fire into attention. Otherwise, as a species, we wouldn't be here on this planet.

Chronic stress, on the other hand, has a very detrimental role in brain function. Much of it is focused around the hormone cortisol and one of the derivatives of cortisol called tetrahydrodeoxycorticosterone (THDOC). In acute situations, this

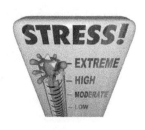

compound has a strong anti-seizure effect. However, in the long-term with chronic stress, the same compound becomes very pro-seizure. So, stress is a major trigger of both headaches and seizures. This is most likely due to this particular hormone.

So, it all boils back down to needing to manage our stress with a variety of different tools to keep stress levels under control. Ideally, any stress we experience is the short-term brain protective stress rather than the long-term chronic brain damaging stress.

ADRENAL FATIGUE

The health of the adrenal glands is another strong factor affecting the level of progesterone that can be converted to allopregnanolone to protect the brain. In mainstream medicine, the adrenal glands did not really share the limelight with other more notorious diseases like cancer, diabetes or osteoporosis. However, if you searched the Pub Med database (the largest repository of medical information on the planet), for the phrase Hypothalamic Pituitary Adrenal axis dysfunction (HPA axis dysfunction, for short), you would find more than 5,000 articles relating stress to almost every disease and condition known to man. HPA access dysfunction is a well-recognized dysfunction in the human body, is incredibly common and affects a variety of diseases today.

This is a very real entity. Typically, if physicians want to evaluate patients' adrenal function, most use blood testing (most often cortisol), giving a single snapshot during the day. However, cortisol levels fluctuate throughout the day, and this can make an accurate assessment difficult because it does not give an idea of the daily fluctuations. Overall, levels should be higher in the morning, slowly tapering down to drop off at the end of the night so that one can go to sleep. Many people have a shifted cortisol rhythm where they're low in the morning – so these people drag – and then they're too high at night -- so they have a hard time falling asleep. Instead of fixing the adrenal function, we take sleep medications to help us sleep. But that hasn't fixed the problem at all, and it will most likely make it worse in the long run. Because of those fluctuations, I feel that the best way to check adrenal hormones is with saliva testing done four times throughout the day.

The adrenal cortex – the outside of the adrenal gland – produces three main hormones. The first is aldosterone, which helps regulate blood pressure. Basically, it helps conserve sodium and keeps our blood pressure up. This may sound strange in today's society. After all, who the heck needs to keep one's blood pressure up? Don't most people have problems with high blood pressure? However, back in the hunter gatherer days, low blood pressure was a much greater concern than was high blood pressure. So the body has a mechanism in place to bring up blood pressure, but no mechanism is in place to take down the blood pressure.

The other hormone that the adrenal cortex produces is dehydroepiandrosterone (DHEA). This is the hormone that goes on to produce testosterone, estrogen and progesterone in both males and females. Both sexes produce DHEA, but the production is obviously at different levels.

The third hormone the adrenal cortex produces is cortisol, the body's stress hormones. Cortisol does wonderful things – when it is part of a healthy body response to stress. However, as previously mentioned, chronic stress really wreaks havoc on our bodies, and we start to produce elevated levels of cortisol.

When we beat our adrenal glands up too much from chronic stress, something called the pregnanolone steal occurs. In essence, the adrenal cortex only has so much precursor "stuff" to work with. When the body is stressed, all of those resources go towards making cortisol, and the production of the other two hormones starts to drop. So one gets lower levels of aldosterone and lower levels of DHEA. With lower levels of aldosterone, a person is going to have a problem keeping blood pressure up. That's why people who are experiencing adrenal insufficiency may actually have low blood pressure and crave salt. It is the body's attempt to make up for the lowered levels of aldosterone.

Of course, if you let it go long enough, the cortisol that's being produced will start to negatively affect other bodily systems and create elevated blood pressure.

When it comes to protecting the brain, the major problem with adrenal fatigue is the reduced levels of DHEA. Less DHEA mean less of the hormones that we need, including the progesterone needed to be converted to allopregnanolone.

Overall, managing stress is an absolutely integral component for a variety of different reasons to improve your brain health. Unfortunately, once one begins to manage stress, some peoples' adrenal glands are not able to recover to the level of optimal function because they have just been too beaten up for too long. In that case, there are a variety of adrenal support formulas available from physicians who understand their use. We have had great success with using these types of supplements to improve patients' adrenal function.

CHAPTER TEN SUMMARY AND ACTION STEPS

Summary:

1. Menstrual migraines typically occur in the last half of the menstrual cycle (day 21-28). This can be a result of lowered levels of iron and iron supplementation can, in some cases, produce very strong results.

2. Progesterone gets converted to a compound called allopregnanolone. Allopregnanolone is one of the most potent brain protective compounds on the planet. Our adrenal glands play a role in the production of progesterone in the body. Because of this, make sure your adrenal glands are functioning properly. Stress contributes to adrenal dysfunction.

3. Being prediabetic drastically affects the health of a woman's ovarian function, lowering the production and release of progesterone. For that reason, maintaining an anti-diabetic lifestyle is of critical importance.

4. Short-term stress actually protects the brain very well, but chronic stress is one of the most damaging factors to our brain health.

Action Steps:
1. If you experience menstrual migraines, add 10-15 mg of iron for two weeks beginning on day 14 of your cycle.
2. If you consider yourself a stress monster, pay careful attention to Chapter 11, titled Calming the Brain, for tools to help you manage your stress. If you have concerns about the health of your adrenal glands, testing is simple and can give you an idea of how your adrenals are working. Check the resources section for labs that do adrenal testing. If there is a problem, many supplements are available to improve adrenal function.
3. Adopting a pre-diabetic lifestyle is critical for all aspects of health. Check the resources section for more information on the required lifestyle changes.

In Chapter 11, since stress is so damaging to the brain, we will begin to look at tools to help you manage your stress. This will include devices that can help you control the damage stress does to your brain

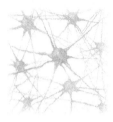

CALMING
THE BRAIN

Chapter 11

There are a lot of ways to calm the brain and keep one neuron from inappropriately firing to its unsuspecting neighbor. We have already mentioned some of them, like exercise, nutrition and supplementation.

MEDITATION

Arguably one of the most powerful methods to calm the brain, a way that has been around for several thousand years, is meditation. Meditation can be as complex as a full-blown transcendental meditation course or can be as simple as a relaxation CD that you can buy used at a bookstore for $5. Everyone has to pick what's going to work best for him or her.

Meditation has been shown to actually calm the brain. This is based on electroencephalagram (EEG) studies where less brain activity was present during meditation. Realize that there is no other time when the brain truly quiets down. Even in sleep, the brain remains very active. Only during meditation do we see brain waves and brain activity slow down. Because of those benefits, meditation can be a powerful tool for improving brain function in a positive way.

BIOFEEDBACK

Biofeedback is a procedure where a patient is hooked up to a device that monitors some aspect of the body, such as heart rate, breathing rate, body temperature or blood pressure. These aspects are then tied to measurable feedback such as a higher or lower audio tone, a dancing spot on a computer monitor or colors on a monitor.

There is actually a device called the RESPeRATE, which is FDA-approved to lower blood pressure and is basically a biofeedback device for breathing. The device works by putting on headphones and listening to the tones that indicate when to breathe in and when to breathe out. During this time period, you find that your focus is entirely on your breathing. Once that happens, you're not focusing on anything else, which is essentially a form of meditation that allows the brain to quiet down. In our office, we've had people who are in the middle of an anxiety attack use the RESPeRATE. In 15 minutes, they are a completely relaxed person.

There are other devices similar to the RESPeRATE. One uses visual stimuli where you focus on certain designs with specific music playing in the background, and you find that the focus on what you are hearing and seeing becomes so intense that it gives the brain a chance to rest and not think about everything else that contributes to your stress levels.

We live in a society that imposes stresses on us that are beyond anything that any society has ever come across before. It is at work. It is at home. These stressors don't ever seem to go away. Our body deals real well with acute stress, but it is the chronic stress that really starts to break down our brains.

These tools and others can help to calm your brain, but you also need to take a good look at your life and what is stressing you and do whatever it takes to start to remove the stresses or learn to let them go. Quite frankly, whatever you're stressing about today, and probably the next 10 things you're going to stress about tomorrow, really aren't going to matter. They're going to happen whether or not you stress about them. However, we seem to stress more about the things that are most out of our control. Does this not seem ridiculous? If they're out of our control, what's the point of stressing over them? And, there is no doubt that your stress levels are destroying your brain slowly, piece by agonizing piece.

THE IMPORTANCE OF SLEEP

While our conscious mind may not be alert while sleeping, this does not mean that our brain is inactive during this time. Far from it. But sleep is not important because it allows your brain to relax, but rather because processing and healing occurs during sleep that we do not yet fully understand. However, it is clear that lack of sleep is a strong trigger for those suffering from migraines and seizures. For that reason, getting a good night's sleep is essential for good brain health.

This task is not always as easy as it sounds. As mentioned, stress hormones like cortisol should be higher in the morning and lower at night, allowing our brains to slide into restorative sleep. Stress throws off this rhythm, leading to higher cortisol levels at night, making sleep nearly impossible.

A mistake at this point would be to step in with pharmaceutical intervention such as Valium or other sedatives, Ambien or Lunestra. Not only is the effectiveness of these drugs questionable, but they do absolutely nothing to fix the underlying problem creating the sleep disturbance.

The long-term solution to sleep problems is stress management and exercise. Few things will restore a healthy sleep pattern as well as these two. In the short term, natural compounds like valerian root may be effective on an individual basis to calm the brain enough to allow sleep to occur naturally. Melatonin, the hormone mentioned earlier, may also help to restore normal sleep patterns. Typically, start dosages at .5 mg an hour or so before the desired bedtime.

CHAPTER 11 SUMMARY AND ACTION STEPS

Summary:

1. There is no question that stress and its effect on the brain is one of the most damaging factors involved in brain health.

2. Protecting from and eliminating stress in our lives needs to be the utmost priority if you hope to achieve good brain health.

3. Achieving a restful night's sleep is critical to good brain health.

Action Steps:

1. Find a meditative tool that will work for you. This can include prayer, certain forms of yoga, Transcendental Meditation or some other stress relief technique. Consider the Natural Stress Relief provided in the resources section.

2. If you find one of the above techniques very difficult to perform (it is common for those whose brains are on "overdrive" to not be able to perform meditation effectively because their brains will not "shut down," as ironic as that may sound) consider finding some type of biofeedback device such as the RESPeRATE. See the resources section for more information.

3. If sleeping is a problem, consider valerian root, melatonin or some type of soothing activity before bed to calm yourself. Aromatherapy baths, relaxing walks or reading may help.

PARTING WORDS

As mentioned early on, none of the advice in this book is designed to replace a current medicinal program. Going off of medications abruptly is, in most cases, a very, very bad idea. Imagine driving a car with both the gas and the brake pressed to the floor. Quickly come off of the brake and see what happens. It's not going to be pretty.

Evaluate the aspects in this book you know you can adapt easily and make the changes. Continue to add positive changes as you are ready. Discuss these changes with your doctor with the ultimate goal of being medication free and brain-healthy.

If you decide that these changes are just "too difficult," then you must accept the fact that your brain will continue on its slow decline into poorer and poorer function, accompanied by loss of cognitive function and a much greater risk of stroke and heart disease.

However, I sincerely hope that this book has had an impact on your decisions. Given the time you have spent reading this book, my wish for you is that you will begin to implement changes in your life and improve your brain health and will not be a statistic.

To your long-term brain health...

RESOURCES

BAHADORI LEANNESS PROGRAM

http://www.leanness-steps.com/000000996e0b0410e/index.
html

KETOGENIC DIET

http://en.wikipedia.org/wiki/Ketogenic_diet
http://www.dietketogenic.com/index.php
http://www.charliefoundation.org/
http://www.matthewsfriends.org/

ELIMINATION DIET

http://integrativemedicine.arizona.edu/file/11270/handout_
elimination_diet_patient.pdf

http://www.functionalmedicine.org/content_management/
files/ifm_Comp_Elim_Diet_091503.pdf
http://www.cfids.org/archives/1998/pre-1999-article01.asp

VITAMIN D RESOURCES
http://www.vitamindcouncil.org/
http://www.umm.edu/altmed/articles/vitamin-d-000340.htm

AROMATHERAPY
http://www.youngliving.com/en_US/index.html

ANTI-DIABETIC LIFESTYLE
http://lifecarechiropractic.com/blog/general-information/
recommendations/

STRESS MANAGEMENT
http://lifecarechiropractic.com/blog/general-information/
product-reviews/resperate-reviews-and-cuts-down-stress-in-
15-minutes/
http://www.natural-stress-relief.com/stress/wellbeing.htm

REFERENCES

1. http://www.sciencedirect.com/science?_ob=ArticleURL&_
   udi=B6WDT-4PSJT38-1&_user=10&_
   coverDate=11%2F30%2F2007&_rdoc=1&_fmt=&_
   orig=search&_sort=d&view=c&_acct=C000050221&_
   version=1&_urlVersion=0&_userid=10&md5=e09cf10bd8
   096ee931829742ac8a4ca6

2. http://www.sciencedirect.com/science?_ob=ArticleURL&_
   udi=B6T34-51S0D3K-1&_user=3211203&_
   coverDate=02%2F28%2F2011&_rdoc=1&_
   fmt=high&_orig=search&_origin=search&_sort=d&_
   docanchor=&view=c&_acct=C000050221&_version=1&_
   urlVersion=0&_userid=3211203&md5=99ffe56658378ca
   634edfa92b18dc6ff&searchtype=a

3. http://www.jmptonline.org/article/S0161-4754(11)00068-6/abstract

4. http://onlinelibrary.wiley.com/doi/10.1111/j.1526-4610.2006.00684.x/abstract;jsessionid=0FE0594A17A599 94E0CF35F68B6C7E12.d02t01

5. Neuromolecular Med. 2002;2(2):215-31

6. Free Rad Bio Med. 2004; 1951-62

7. (http://ehp03.niehs.nih.gov/article/fetchArticle.action?articleURI=info%3Adoi%2F10.1289%2Fehp.118-a217a)

8. http://ehp03.niehs.nih.gov/article/fetchArticle.action?articleURI=info%3Adoi%2F10.1289%2Fehp.0901757#Environmental Mercury Methylation

9. Prog Neuropsychopharmacol Biol Psychiatry. 2004 Aug;28(5):771-99

10. http://jn.physiology.org/cgi/content/abstract/57/2/496

11. Trends Pharmacol Sci. 1998 Aug;19(8):328-34

12. J Physiol Biochem. 2003 Jun;59(2):129-41

13. Int J Mol Med. 2004 Jun;13(6):873-6

14. Ann Neurol, 1992 Feb; 31(2):119-30

15. Neuromolecular Med, 2003;3(2):65-94

16. J Neurochem. 11998 Dec;71(6):2392-400

17. Science. 1993 Oct 29;262(5134):689-95

18. Biomed Pharmacother. 2004 Jan;58(1):39-46

19. http://www.biomedcentral.com/1472-6823/9/3/abstract

20. http://www.medical-hypotheses.com/article/S0306-9877(06)00737-7/abstract

21. http://www.ncbi.nlm.nih.gov/pubmed/11903088

22. http://www.ncbi.nlm.nih.gov/pubmed/10479881

23. http://www.ncbi.nlm.nih.gov/pubmed/2909707

24. http://www.ncbi.nlm.nih.gov/pubmed/20647174

25. http://jcem.endojournals.org/cgi/content/full/89/4/1641

26. http://www.ncbi.nlm.nih.gov/pubmed/8598704

27. http://www.neurology.org/content/78/18/1401.abstract

28. http://www.nature.com/emboj/journal/v19/n8/
    abs/7593005a.html

29. Neuroscience. 1996 Jul;73(1):185-200

30. J Neurochem. 1995 May;64(5):2239-47

31. Epilepsy Research. 1998 April;30(2):153-158

32. Neuroscience. 1996 Apr; 71(4):1043-8

33. Indian J Physiol Pharmacol. 2003 Oct;47(4):373-86

34. http://www.sciencedirect.com/science/article/pii/
    S0304394098007903

35. http://www.sciencedirect.com/science/article/pii/
    S1525505011003866

36. http://www.if-pan.krakow.pl/pjp/pdf/2011/1_1_ab.pdf

37. http://informahealthcare.com/doi/
    abs/10.1517/13543784.15.4.367

38. http://www.sciencedirect.com/science/article/pii/
    S0920121111001689

39. Seligmann H, et al. *Am J Med* 1991 Aug;91(2):151-155

40. http://www.pnas.org/content/92/8/3124.full.pdf+html

41. http://www.ncbi.nlm.nih.gov/pubmed/15056857

42. http://www.seizure-journal.com/article/S1059-
    1311(03)00161-4/abstract

43. http://www.neurology.org/cgi/content/abstract/45/9/1660

GLOSSARY

ATP – Adenosine Triphosphate – the "energy currency" of the cell. This is the molecule that our cells use to get things done.

GABA (gamma-aminobutyric acid) – a neurotransmitter, generally acts to calm down the activity of the brain.

Glutamate – a neurotransmitter, generally acts to speed up the activity of the brain.

Epinephrine – aka adrenaline, a neurotransmitter, generally acts to speed up the activity of the brain.

Free radicals – damaging molecules that can result in the destruction of everything they touch inside of a cell.

Mitochondria – a small piece of machinery inside every cell of our bodies that makes the energy needed for a cell to run properly.

Neurotransmitter – the molecule that our brain cells use to communicate with one another. Examples include serotonin, GABA, epinephrine and dopamine.

Oxidative stress – the situation that occurs when the number of free radicals our body produces is more than our body can fight off.

Phytonutrients – compounds that are produced by plants that help to protect our health in some way when we eat these foods.